NEW WAYS TO HEALTH

A GUIDE TO CHIROPRACTIC

Susan Moore   DC

in association with The British
Chiropractic Association

HAMLYN

Series editor Hal Robinson of
Clark Robinson Limited, London

First published 1988 by the Hamlyn Publishing
Group Limited, a division of
the Octopus Publishing Group,
Michelin House, 81 Fulham Road,
London SW3 6RB

ISBN 0 600 56016 3

Printed by Mandarin Offset in Hong Kong

Editorial Note
He or she. We have followed the sex of the
author and the practitioner in the photographs
when frequent referral to the chiropractor is
necessary in the text. Of course the profession is
open to both sexes.

JACM

A GUIDE TO
CHIROPRACTIC

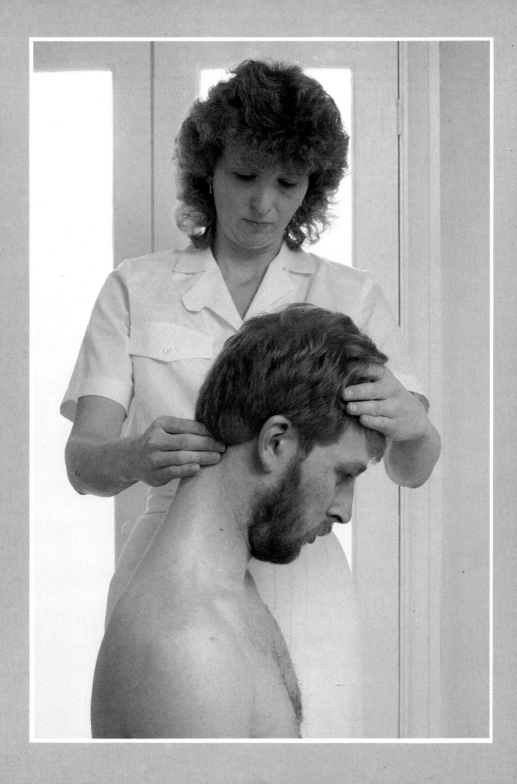

CONTENTS

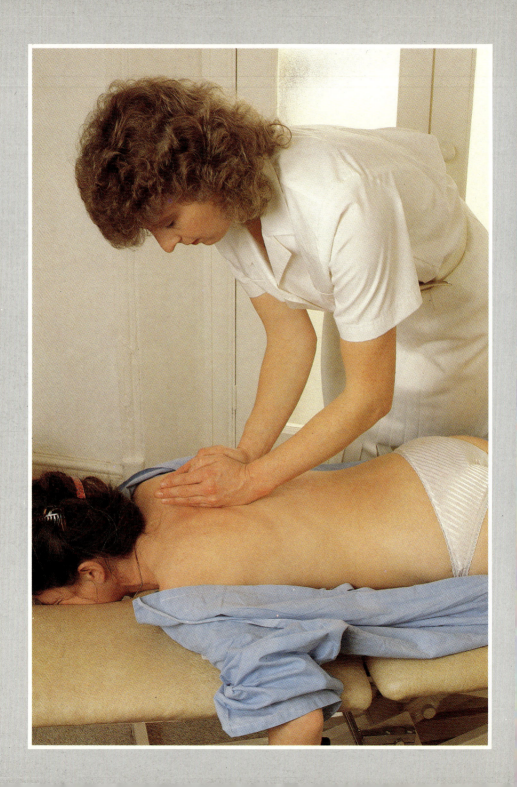

1

INTRODUCTION

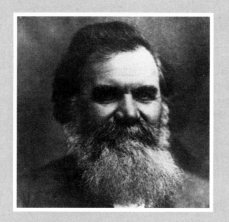

The healing art of chiropractic is a comparatively new science that looks both to the future and to the past. It sees the future of health care in terms of sensitive and integrated therapy, yet draws on the past, where evidence of successful healing based on similar principles to those employed by chiropractors today is abundant.

In the latter part of the twentieth century we enjoy standards of health that are in general higher than ever before. Yet in our search for perfection we are finding fault increasingly with the established medical system that is so successful at eradicating disease, yet seems ill-equipped to promote positive health.

The approach of chiropractors to health is positive from the outset. Their assumption that good health is our natural state encourages them to look first at the whole person, to see what may have gone wrong, and then to look for ways to correct this. Their objectives focus on the spine and its nerves, because to a chiropractor these are the centre of our physical being.

Chiropractic today

Chiropractic is best understood by recognizing at the outset that it has two potentially contradictory aspects. It is quite accurate to describe it as both an art and a science. Modern chiropractors are fully conversant with orthodox medical science and also use orthodox methods in their diagnosis of conditions. This scientific approach is complemented, however, by the chiropractor's art, which lies in the use of the hands to detect minute changes of spinal function and to correct those changes using refined techniques of spinal adjustment or manipulation.

A chiropractor treats a great variety of disorders. Most common among these are problems related to the muscles and joints, which include common conditions such as back pain, neck pain, disc problems and arthritis. The intimate connections between spinal irritation and organic problems such as digestive, respiratory or even gynaecological disorders are not overlooked, however, and many such conditions still respond to chiropractic manipulation. Chiropractic is a particularly valuable therapy where orthodox treatment with drugs has failed.

Chiropractic and orthodox medicine

Manipulation is not the exclusive preserve of chiropractors. Osteopathy, which has interesting similarities but also important differences to chiropractic, uses manipulation. Manipulation is also practised by a few doctors in the field of orthodox medicine. There are, however, far too few practitioners within the orthodox field to satisfy demand, so it has been left to the chiropractors to build and develop this particular area of expertise as their own.

The reasons for this seem to be that, in many ways, orthodox medicine has lost its roots. Surgery, drugs and technology have provided it with its huge successes and have made it a science of the future as much as of the present. In its triumphant progress, however, it seems to have left many people behind. Most neglected are those who are ill or in pain without obvious cause. In particular, anyone suffering from a condition, such as back pain, that may be chronically troublesome but is not life-threatening, all too commonly finds that orthodox treatment cannot help. Neither technology, drugs nor surgery seem to have the answer.

In the great majority of cases it is circumstances of this type that encourage patients to consult a chiropractor. They do not want a drug that will simply mask their symptoms. They want to know the cause of their pain and they want that cause corrected. Happily, by using a combination of scientific knowledge and the art of manipulation, more often than not the chiropractor is able to help them.

The Founder of chiropractic

Chiropractic emerged as one of the successful medical discoveries of the second half of the nineteenth century. It developed in the United States at about the same time as osteopathy as a result of research and experimentation by Daniel David Palmer, who carried out his first formal chiropractic manipulation in 1895. Although his approach to conventional medical science has been described as eccentric, Palmer was in fact well-read in both anatomy and physiology, devoting much time to the study of the spine and how it worked, eventually concluding that disease was the result of abnormal spinal function.

His students and followers have learned his techniques, studied his methods and refined his theoretical approach to bring the science of chiropractic to its present state. At the same time, they have concentrated in their training on learning his healing, manipulative, 'chiropractic' art, so that all aspects of his healing skills have been retained for the benefit of chiropractors and their patients today.

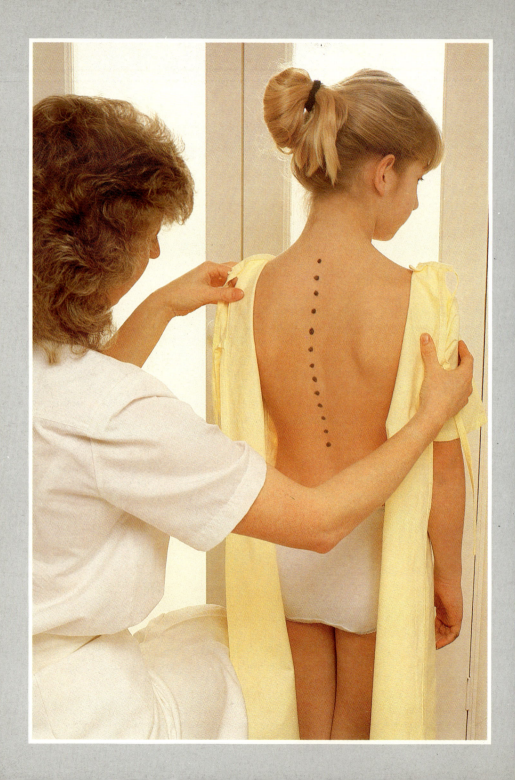

2

HOW CAN CHIROPRACTIC HELP?

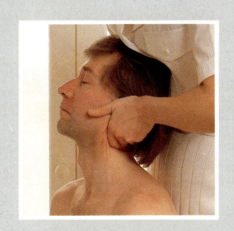

The human body is an extremely complex biological machine in which overall co-ordination and control lie with the brain, spinal cord and their associated nerves. All the functions of the body are governed, in one way or another, by the activities of the brain, which receives information and transmits instructions by means of the nervous system. In everyday life, we are totally unaware that this process is continually happening. For instance, when you turn the pages of this book, your brain sends instructions to the muscles in your hands and arms, and co-ordinates the fine movements required to hold and manipulate the pages.

The spinal cord lies in a bony canal running through the middle of the bones (vertebrae) that make up the spine. Because of this proximity of the spine and spinal cord, chiropractors believe that alteration to normal spinal function and mobility affects the transmission of nerve impulses along the spinal cord and spinal nerves. This, in turn, then affects the parts of the body served by the nerves. If the nerves that are irritated serve one of the internal organs, eventually the irritation could result in some sort of disorder in that organ. On the other hand, if the nerves that are irritated supply muscles and soft tissues, the result may be a referred pain, such as the pain felt in an arm or a leg from pressure on a nerve in the neck or low part of the back. To understand how this happens, it will help to know something about the structure and function of the spine and nervous system.

Body and spine Many people are totally unaware of how complex their bodies are until they go wrong in some way. This is especially true of spine and back pain. Many back pain sufferers find it difficult to understand initially how a back problem is caused or how the relationship between the spine and the nerves can cause referred pain in the legs or arms.

The spine

The spine, or spinal column, is a complicated bony structure made up of the spine itself and its vertebrae, and the various nerves, discs, muscles and ligaments associated with it. All these 'elements' affect the correct functioning of the spine.

The spine consists of 24 individual vertebrae, made up of 7 in the neck (the cervical vertebrae), 12 in the upper back (thoracic vertebrae) and 5 in the lower back (lumbar vertebrae). Attached to the base of the spine are five vertebrae fused together to form the sacrum. And attached to the base of the sacrum are three more fused vertebrae called the coccyx, or tail bone. The skull pivots on the first cervical vertebra at the top of the neck.

When a normal spine is viewed from the back, it appears to be straight. When viewed from the side, it has the shape of an elongated letter S. In a normal spine, three distinct curves can be seen. The first, in the neck, curves inwards towards the

THE STRUCTURE OF THE SPINE

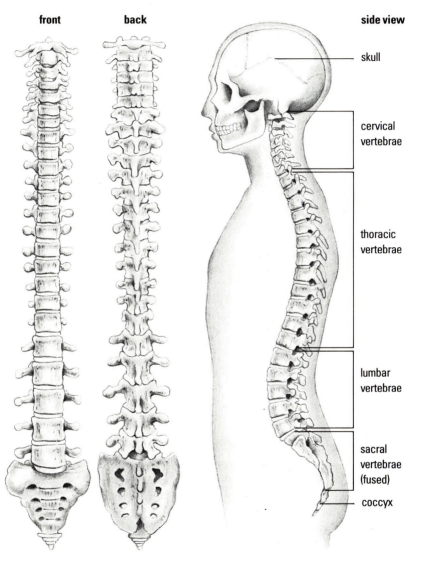

front   back   side view

skull

cervical
vertebrae

thoracic
vertebrae

lumbar
vertebrae

sacral
vertebrae
(fused)

coccyx

Seen from the front or back, the normal spine should be straight, with no sideways curves. When viewed from the side, three distinct curves become visible: one inward curve in the neck (the cervical lordosis*); one outward curve in the upper back (the* thoracic kyphosis*), and one inward curve in the lower back (the* lumbar lordosis*).*

curves inwards towards the front; it is known as the cervical lordosis. The second, in the upper back, curves outwards and is known as the thoracic kyphosis. The third, in the lower back, curves inwards once again; it is called the lumbar lordosis.

These curves are essential for the spine to function normally and to reduce the effect of stress and wear and tear. The cervical curve on the top of the spine helps to cushion the weight of the skull. In some people the curves are exaggerated or reduced, and this tends to cause stress areas which can eventually result in back pain.

The spine acts as an attachment for the 12 pairs of ribs in the upper back. Some of the ribs are also attached to the breastbone, or sternum, at the front. The spine is linked to the arms through the bones of the shoulders and to the legs through the pelvic bones.

The shoulders consist of the two shoulder blades (scapulae) at the back, which articulate with the arms at the sides and with the collar bones (clavicles) at the front. The collar bones are in turn jointed with the breastbone. By this means, the rib cage is linked to the spine and the arms.

The pelvis consists of the two large pelvic bones, which are jointed to the sacrum at the back and with each other in the front to form the pubic bone. The pelvic bones also form the sockets for the hip joints on each side – thus attaching the pelvis to the legs.

The skeleton therefore forms the basic scaffolding of the body, on which the rest is built.

The brain and spinal cord

One of the chief functions of the skull is to house the very delicate brain, and a main function of the spine is to surround and protect the equally delicate spinal cord. The spinal cord arises from the base of the brain, and travels down inside the spinal column to its base. Branching out from the spinal cord are the spinal nerves, which supply the various parts of the body such as the internal organs and the muscles.

The spinal nerves arise from each side of the spinal cord between the vertebrae. Once they have left the spine, some of the nerve roots join together again to form a nerve plexus, from which they travel to various parts of the body. In the cervical region, the collection of nerve roots is known as the cervical plexus; in the sacral region it is known as the sacral plexus; and so on.

When back pain starts We can misuse our spines for many years before we actually start to suffer with back pain. Often it is past injuries that finally result in present back pain. Strangely though, different people can show the same degree of wear and tear and injury to the spine, but suffer completely different symptoms and degrees of pain.

THE SKELETON

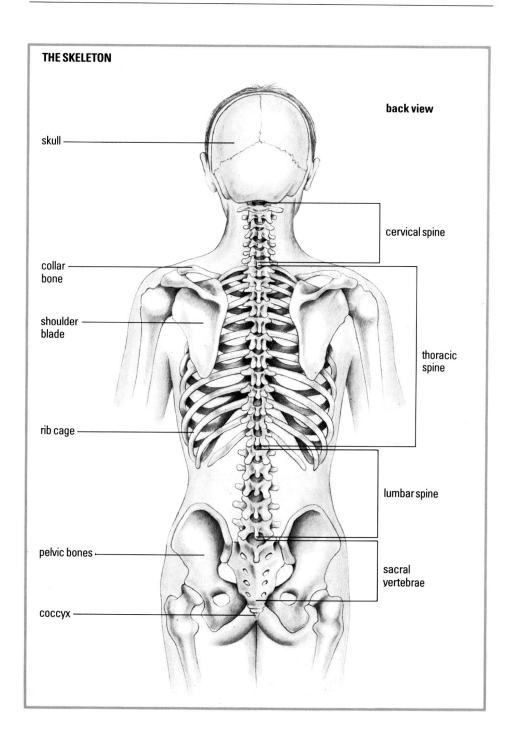

back view

skull

cervical spine

collar bone

shoulder blade

thoracic spine

rib cage

lumbar spine

pelvic bones

sacral vertebrae

coccyx

Sciatica In some cases the person may not suffer with back pain, just pain in the back of the leg as in sciatica. Many people do not realize the connection between the low back and referred pain in the leg. Even though there may be no back pain, it is still necessary to treat the low back to reduce the pressure on the nerves supplying the legs, as these produce the pain.

The base of the spinal cord forms a bundle of nerve branches called the *cauda equina* (Latin for a horses's tail, which it resembles). The end of the spinal cord proper is about level with the first or second lumbar vertebra. The *cauda equina* is made up of many nerve roots, which combine to travel together down the spinal column, leaving the spine at various levels in the lower back.

One of the main nerves arising from the base of the spine, which then travels down the back of each leg, is the sciatic nerve. Irritation high in the sciatic nerve can result in a referred pain in the back of the leg, the condition known as sciatica.

The nervous system

The brain, spinal cord and nerves make up the nervous system. The central nervous system (CNS) is made up of the brain and spinal cord, and constitutes the main control centre and message network for all the body's activities.

The peripheral nervous sytem is made up of the nerves that govern motor and sensory activities. Motor activities are those that are responsible for movement – for example, the movement of an arm, leg, finger or toe. Sensory activities are those in which we respond automatically, as when we remove our hand from a hot cup. They also provide us with our senses, such as sight, hearing, touch, smell and taste. Touch sensors in the skin can distinguish between hot and cold, hard and soft, and so on; others register pain.

The autonomic nervous system is often described as an automatic one because it controls functions of which we are not normally aware, such as breathing. This system is itself further sub-divided into the sympathetic and parasympathetic systems, which produce opposite and equal effects on the body and in this way allow it to maintain a state of equilibrium or balance. For example, when danger threatens the sympathetic system speeds up the heartbeat and slows digestion. When the danger is past, the parasympathetic system slows the heartbeat back to normal and speeds up digestion. So the autonomic nervous system controls the involuntary processes of the body.

Through its various branches, the nervous system serves every tissue and organ, and controls its rate and mode of action. It is thus easy to understand that any interruption to this system can have far-reaching and even dramatic effects, not only in obvious symptoms such as pain, but in symptoms expressed in other ways – such as acid indigestion, constipation, diarrhoea, menstrual pains, and so on.

THE CENTRAL NERVOUS SYSTEM

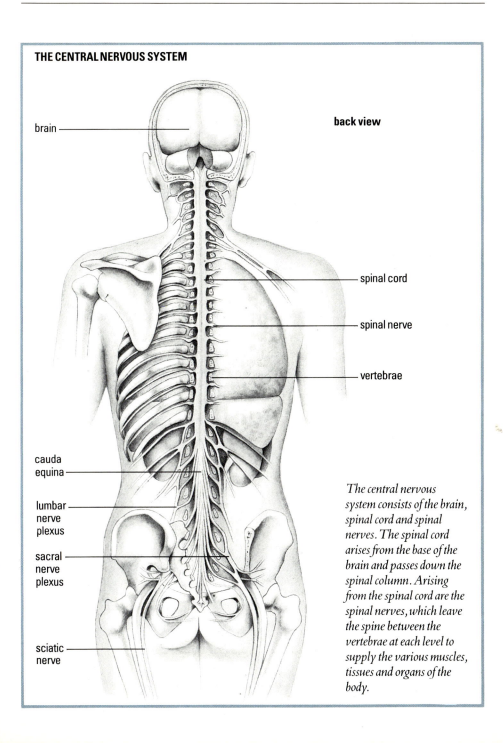

brain

back view

spinal cord

spinal nerve

vertebrae

cauda
equina

lumbar
nerve
plexus

sacral
nerve
plexus

sciatic
nerve

*The central nervous
system consists of the brain,
spinal cord and spinal
nerves. The spinal cord
arises from the base of the
brain and passes down the
spinal column. Arising
from the spinal cord are the
spinal nerves, which leave
the spine between the
vertebrae at each level to
supply the various muscles,
tissues and organs of the
body.*

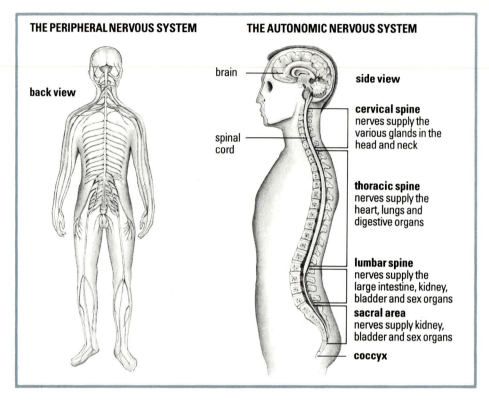

THE PERIPHERAL NERVOUS SYSTEM

back view

THE AUTONOMIC NERVOUS SYSTEM

brain

side view

spinal cord

cervical spine
nerves supply the various glands in the head and neck

thoracic spine
nerves supply the heart, lungs and digestive organs

lumbar spine
nerves supply the large intestine, kidney, bladder and sex organs

sacral area
nerves supply kidney, bladder and sex organs

coccyx

The peripheral nervous system starts from the spinal cord and nerves and passes to the periphery supplying the various parts of the arms, legs, chest and abdomen.

The autonomic nervous system supplies the various organs of the body. It is made up of the sympathetic and parasympathetic systems which have opposite effects on the organs concerned.

Muscles, tendons and ligaments

The human body is covered in layers of muscles which attach the various parts of the body to each other. Many people think that in our back, for instance, there is a covering consisting of one large sheet of muscle. This is not the case. The back is particularly complicated because it is covered by a layer of deep muscles overlaid by a system of superficial ones. The muscles that make up the different layers are of various lengths and run in various directions. Not only do they help to hold the skeleton together, they also allow the different movements of flexion, extension, rotation and sideways bending of the spine and other parts of the body.

At each end, muscles are attached to bones by tendons. Some tendons are very long. For example, long tendons run from the fingers to the muscles in the forearm (which contract to bend and straighten the fingers). To give added support, moveable joints have short fibrous structures called ligaments, which hold the bones in position.

THE MUSCLES OF THE BACK

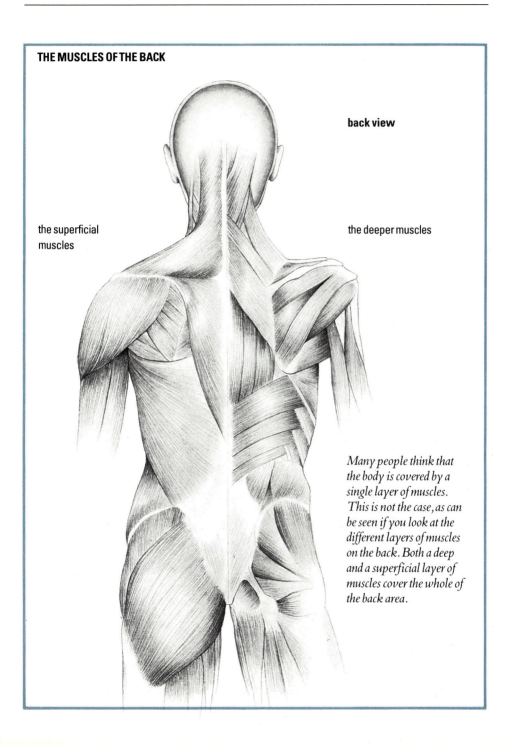

back view

the superficial muscles

the deeper muscles

Many people think that the body is covered by a single layer of muscles. This is not the case, as can be seen if you look at the different layers of muscles on the back. Both a deep and a superficial layer of muscles cover the whole of the back area.

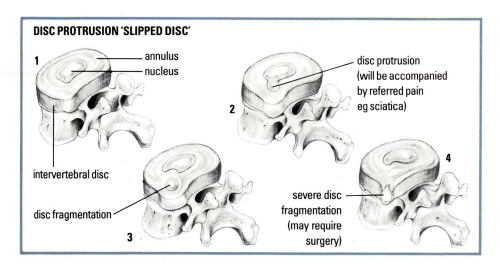

DISC PROTRUSION 'SLIPPED DISC'

1 — annulus — nucleus

intervertebral disc

disc fragmentation

2 — disc protrusion (will be accompanied by referred pain eg sciatica)

4

3 — severe disc fragmentation (may require surgery)

The intervertebral disc (1) consists of an outer layer of ring-like cartilage (the annulus fibrosus) with a more fluid-like centre (the nucleus pulposus). Strain on the disc can often result in a weakening in the outer layers of the cartilage. This allows part of the nucleus to protrude into the outer layers, causing these layers also to protrude.

Disc protrusion will frequently lead to pressure on one of the spinal nerves and result in referred pain such as sciatica (2). In more severe cases, the disc may fragment (3) and part of the disc actually break off (4). This can lead to very severe back and referred pain, and often requires surgery.

Vertebrae

As we have seen, the spine is made up of individual bones called vertebrae. Each vertebra articulates with the one above and below it at a vertebral, or facet, joint. These joints not only link the vertebrae together, but also allow movement of the spine as a whole. At an individual level, each vertebra has to be able to articulate freely with the one next to it.

Intervertebral discs

In addition to the vertebrae and their associated muscles, tendons and ligaments, the spine has its own special structures called intervertebral discs. These lie between the vertebrae and form part of the spinal column. They act as cushions or shock absorbers and help to reduce the stress and strain on the spine that occurs in normal daily activity and movement.

Each disc consists of a very strong outer ring of fibre (the annulus) surrounding a more fluid-like centre or nucleus. Body movement, particularly bending and stretching, alters the pressure exerted on the discs. In extreme cases, too much pressure may cause a disc to bulge (known medically as a prolapse). The jelly-like centre bulges into the outer ring, making part of the disc protrude. This in turn can cause pressure on the spinal cord or, more often, on a spinal nerve. The result is pain in the back, and possibly also referred pain in an arm or a leg (depending on which spinal nerve is affected). The condition is commonly – but inaccurately – called a slipped disc.

HOW THE SPINE IS MADE UP

Looking at a section of the spine, you can see how it is made up. The individual vertebrae are separated by the intervertebral discs. The bones articulate with each other at the back at the facet joints.

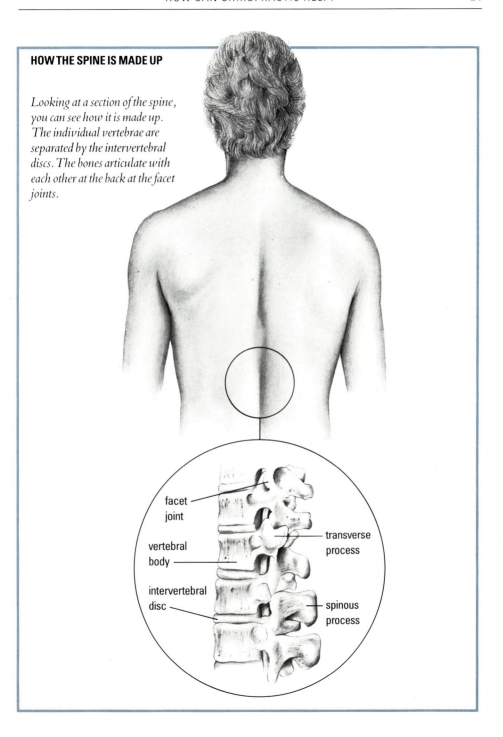

facet joint

transverse process

vertebral body

intervertebral disc

spinous process

The chiropractor's role

It is the job of a chiropractor to detect areas of the spine in which there is restricted or abnormal movement, and to correct any anomalies so that the spine can regain its normal dynamic functions. Any abnormal movement at this level can also cause effects through the nervous system in the form or referred pain in either the musculoskeletal system or internal organs.

The relationship between particular spinal nerves and particular internal organs has been closely studied. A chiropractor frequently encounters cases in which correction of a spinal disorder also relieves other symptoms (such as problems of breathing or digestion). The orthodox medical profession does not readily accept this connection as the basis of a form of treatment – even though the link between the spine and the internal organs is clear – because the mechanism by which the link works is not fully understood. A direct connection is usually accepted only in cases of extreme spinal nerve or spinal cord damage – for example, when a low back injury causes spinal cord damage which results in bladder incontinence. (In an extreme case such as this, surgery is usually essential.)

The reverse direction in this link is also evident. Irritation from an internal organ can produce referred pain which is felt in the spine, shoulder or arm. Such examples include mid-back pain from stomach irritation, right-shoulder pain from liver irritation, and left-arm pain in certain heart complaints. A blocked or inflamed gall bladder is also well known as a cause of referred pain in many different areas of the skeletal system.

It is because of this interrelationship between the nervous system and the function of the internal organs that a chiropractor regards the spine as being so important in the maintenance of good health. Correct biomechanical function of the spine is therefore essential not only for treating musculoskeletal complaints, which is the main role of the chiropractor, but also for the maintenance of ordinary good health from the whole-body or holistic point of view.

It is important to stress, however, that although chiropractors find their skills can benefit a patient in many different ways, they do tend to concentrate mainly on treating musculoskeletal conditions, because these respond particularly well to manipulative therapy. Rheumatism, fibrositis, lumbago and neuralgia are all common but vague terms that describe

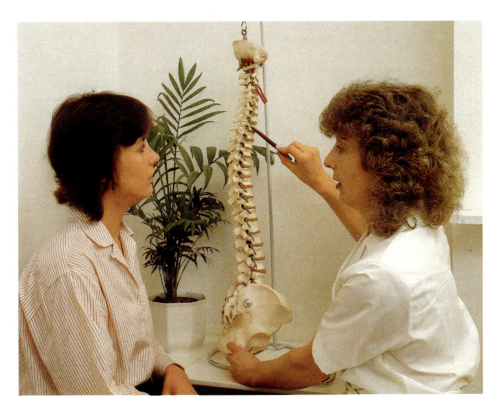

muscular pain – especially pain in the back or joints. The term rheumatism tends to be used when the patient aches all over, fibrositis when there is muscle tension in the neck and shoulders, lumbago for low back pain, and neuralgia for a nerve pain. A chiropractor aims to find the cause of such symptoms and then treat the patient accordingly.

Many people tend to think that chiropractors deal only with back problems. It is also usually thought that back sufferers are middle-aged, overweight and unfit. Neither of these statements is true, as we shall see.

The chiropractor will explain the likely cause of the patient's back pain before treatment begins. Helping the patient to understand her back and how and where it goes wrong will help her to prevent the problem recurring in the future.

Low back pain

Quite a large proportion of patients who consult a chiropractor (an average of 55 per cent), suffer from some sort of low back problem. The causes, however, are many and varied. Alterations to normal spine movements can result in a loss of spinal joint mobility (hypomobility) in an area, with or without irritation of the nerve roots. This can be felt simply as

Bending the back and lifting or twisting without bending the knees is a frequent cause of back pain. Adults are not nearly so flexible as children and so need to take much more care to prevent serious back problems. After pregnancy a mother's spine and pelvis can be especially susceptible to problems when she bends incorrectly, and so it is very important that the mother returns to physical fitness as soon as possible in order to minimize the problem.

back pain, or as referred pain – with pins and needles and even numbness in one or both legs. As already mentioned, referred pain that goes down the back of a leg along the path of the sciatic nerve is known as sciatica. However, other nerves can also be affected; for example, nerve pain that sends pain down the front of the thigh to the knee is called femoral neuralgia. Femoral and sciatic nerves leave the spine at different levels and they are not usually both affected at the same time. A chiropractor will seek to restore normal spinal mobility by using manipulation. This helps to take the pressure off a restricted nerve and allows it to heal, so that eventually the symptoms subside.

The opposite condition also occurs, in which the spinal joints have increased mobility (hypermobility), causing discomfort in the back through excessive soft-tissue pain. This can also be relieved by chiropractic treatment.

Disc problems

The low back is the area of the spine in which disc problems most commonly occur. These are often called 'slipped discs', but this term gives the impression that the whole disc moves

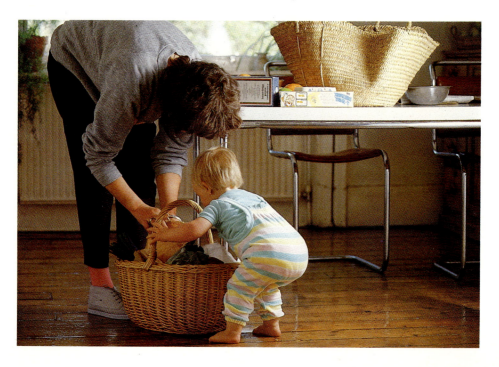

WHY PEOPLE CONSULT A CHIROPRACTOR

Percentage of consultations

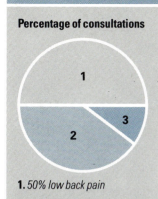

1. *50% low back pain*

2. *40% head, neck and chest pain*

3. *10% extremity joint and other problems*

Low back pain
Low back and leg pain · Sciatica
disc problems · Spinal stenosis,
Fibrositis · Rheumatism
Arthritis · Spondylosis · Spondylitis
Scoliosis · Muscular problems
Hip pain

Extremity joint problems
Tennis elbow · Golfer's elbow,
Problems with hands and wrists
feet and ankles
knees and cartilage

Head, neck and chest pain
Migraine · Tension headaches,
Facial pain
Neck (cervical) Spondylosis
and spondylitis
Rheumatism · Shoulder pain
'Frozen' shoulder · disc problems,
Rib and chest pain
Muscular problems · Fibrositis

Other reasons
Asthma · Menstrual pain
Digestive disorders

out of position, which as we have already seen is not the case. The disc itself is firmly attached to the vertebrae above and below it. It is the more fluid nucleus of the disc that can move under pressure, causing the outer fibres of the disc to bulge. When this happens, the bulge may press on a spinal nerve and cause referred pain in the leg. The precise location of the pain depends on which nerve is irritated.

In such cases there is usually loss of normal vertebral mobility at the affected spinal joints, combined with intense muscle spasm. The chiropractor aims to reduce the muscle spasm and restore spinal movement, thus reducing the pressure on the disc so that it goes back into place. In some more severe cases, however, the disc may cause pressure on the spinal cord itself or may even fragment. The pieces of disc may move about, and then surgery is usually the only option.

Spondylosis, spondylolysis and spondylolythesis

It is said that from the age of 25 onwards we start to exhibit symptoms of wear and tear in the spine. This may be worse in some people than in others. Spondylosis is the term usually employed to describe this process of wear and tear. Chiropractors often find that it is associated with areas of stress, where

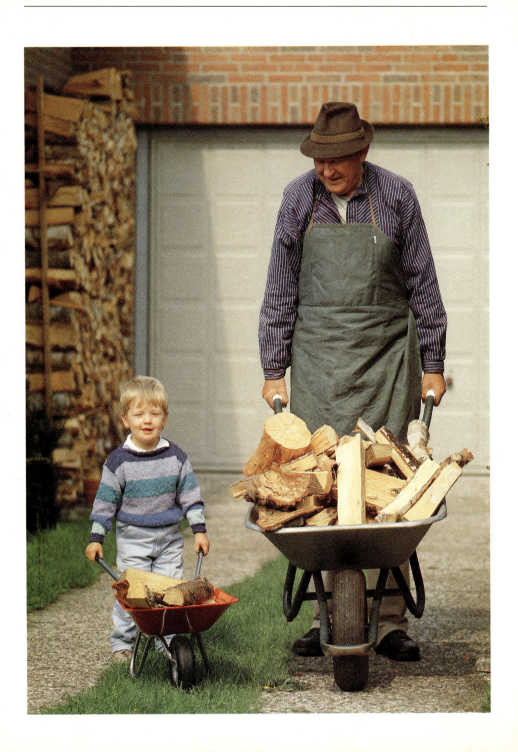

normal spinal mobility is altered in some way. Arthritis is another similar disorder, although when an arthritic condition exists it does not necessarily cause pain. Pain is more often associated with alteration to normal spine movement, and with muscle and soft-tissue spasm.

Spondylolythesis is the name of a condition in which one vertebra moves forward relative to the one below it because of a defect in its structure. It usually affects the low back. Chiropractors frequently treat this condition successfully, and only in very severe cases is surgery required.

Spondylolysis is a similar condition to spondylolythesis; a vertebral defect exists but there is no forward displacement.

Back strains and sprains
It is very easy to strain or sprain the low back and pelvic area. When this happens there is usually intense muscle and ligament spasm and joint fixation. These sorts of conditions can be successfully treated by a chiropractor.

Spinal stenosis
Narrowing of the spinal canal occurs more often than might be expected. The condition is known as spinal stenosis, and it can cause severe low back pain and referred pain in the legs. Reduction of normal vertebral mobility and associated muscle spasm can bring on the symptoms if spinal stenosis already exists in an otherwise healthy person, and many cases respond well to chiropractic treatment. Severe cases, however, often require surgery to enlarge the spinal canal and relieve pressure on the spinal cord. People who do heavy manual work frequently encounter this problem once back trouble arises, and in some industries (such as mining) pre-employment medical checks are carried out to detect any predisposition to back trouble from spinal stenosis.

Muscular problems
Lack of muscle tone and strength in the back, abdominal muscles and thigh muscles can all lead to low back pain. This is because the spine has to rely on other strong muscles – such as those in the legs – to reduce the amount of strain put on the spine itself. A chiropractor is able to reduce any muscle tension in such cases and can advise the patient about exercises to help to tone up and strengthen the appropriate muscles. Referred pain can also arise from sensitive trigger points in the muscles, and these can be relieved using chiropractic treatment.

Backstrain Working in a continual bent or twisted position easily strains the low back and is a common problem in keen gardeners and manual workers such as carpet fitters, electricians and plumbers.

Gardening is a common cause of back problems, from the simple muscular ache to the more severe disc problems. Spring time gardeners are especially susceptible to problems after a winter of little or no exercise. The first dig of the season frequently results in a crop of acute back problems.

Neck pain

The second most common reason that people seek chiropractic care is for treatment of neck problems. As in the low back, loss of normal spinal mobility in the neck area can result in pain, possibly also causing pressure on nerve roots. In such a case any nerve pressure results in referred pain in the arm; numbness or the tingling effect called 'pins and needles' may also occur. Depending on the nerve affected, the pain may be referred to the scalp and face as a type of neuralgia. Chiropractic therapy can help to restore normal mobility and reduce pressure on the nerves, thus relieving the symptoms.

Disc problems can also occur in the neck, in a similar way to the low back, although they are much rarer. Chiropractors can successfully treat some cervical disc problems.

Headaches and migraine may also be related to neck problems and loss of spinal mobility. By restoring normal movement to the spine, the chiropractor is able to reduce pressure on the nerves and relieve the patient's symptoms.

The neck area is frequently affected by muscle tension, caused either by muscle fatigue or the affects of psychological stress and tension. This can result in neck pain, pain across the shoulders, headaches or migraine, or even referred pain in the arms. Relief of the muscle tension by chiropractic treatment can help to reduce these painful symptoms.

It is now known that the jaw joint can be responsible for various types of facial pain, which may radiate into the neck and shoulders. Excessive chewing of gum, ill-fitting dentures and even overstretching the mouth at the dentist can all lead to strain at the jaw joints. Pain is not often felt in the jaw itself, but is usually referred elsewhere – such as the neck pain or the headaches already mentioned. Occasionally the patient is aware only of a certain amount of 'clicking' in the jaw. The chiropractor can examine the jaw and treat it, if necessary, while treating the neck and other areas as well.

The upper back

Pain is also fairly common in the upper back, or thoracic area (the part of the spine opposite the chest). The most frequent site is on the spine between the shoulder blades. The cause can be muscular, with associated loss of normal spinal mobility. Sometimes the ribs are also involved. In severe cases a referred pain may arise as pain in the ribs or an intercostal neuralgia. This is pain that travels along the nerves in the intercostal spaces between the ribs. It may spread all the way round to the

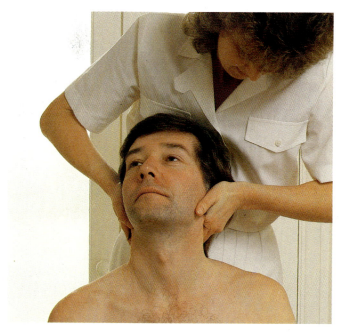

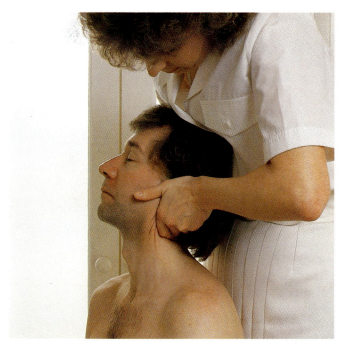

Adjusting the vertebrae in the neck (cervical spine) will help to restore normal joint mobility, relieve muscle spasm and reduce any pressure on the nerves. As a result, pain is minimized and the cause of the problem can be treated.

Patients are often nervous at first about having their necks treated, fearing that it will be a painful experience. However, once they gain confidence in their chiropractor, they relax and find that the treatment is not at all frightening or painful. Here the patient is having his neck adjusted for neck or neck and arm pain.

front of the chest, and may sometimes be mistaken for a chest or heart disorder.

Fortunately disc problems in the upper back area are extremely rare. Fractures of the vertebrae in this area, on the other hand, are more common than fractures of vertebrae in the neck or low back. The cause is usually trauma of some kind, such as injury resulting from an accident.

Spontaneous vertebral fractures sometimes occur in women after the menopause because of alterations to the normal calcium balance in the bones. Although bones get thinner as we get older, not everyone suffers from spinal fractures. Chiropractors cannot treat the fractured bone itself, but they can treat the areas above and below it, and the intense muscle spasm that results from the fracture. In this way they can help to speed recovery.

Anyone can develop the condition known as 'golfer's' or 'tennis' elbow but keen golf and tennis players are most susceptible. This condition (which produces a severe inflammatory reaction around the elbow joint) often responds well to chiropractic treatment. Many professional golfers also suffer from low back problems due to the strain on the spine while playing.

The extremity joints

Apart from the spine, chiropractors also treat other joints, such as the hip, shoulder, knee, ankle and elbow. The most common type of hip problem is an arthritic hip. Many of these require surgery, and the operation for a hip replacement has an extremely high success rate. Not everyone can get surgical treatment exactly when they want it, however. The waiting lists for surgery are frequently long, the hip may not yet be bad enough to justify surgery, or the patient may not be able to undergo surgery for various other medical reasons. In these cases chiropractic treatment can help to reduce the amount of pain and disability. Frequently the pain is felt not only in the hip, but also in the groin and down the front of the thigh. In many cases this can also be relieved.

The shoulder joint takes the brunt of many different injuries – from sport, accidents or unaccustomed repetitive use as in washing windows or decorating. The shoulder is a complicated joint and can take longer to respond to treatment than others. The shoulder condition most frequently seen by chiropractors is a 'frozen shoulder', otherwise known as adhesive capsulitis. This is an inflammation of the capsule around the joint, usually accompanied by severe muscle tension in the joint area. Chiropractic soft-tissue techniques and mobilization can help the healing process.

'Tennis' or 'golfer's' elbow describes severe pain in the elbow joint, on one or both sides. And the sufferer does not necessarily have to have played tennis or golf in order to develop the condition. This condition is, in effect, an inflammatory reaction around the bone in the elbow (termed epicondylitis). It is usually extremely painful and in many cases the patient has an associated problem in the lower part of the neck. Chiropractic treatment can generally help relieve this problem.

Knee and ankle problems frequently result from sporting injuries, such as those sustained in running or playing football, and most chiropractors will treat such disorders. An increasing number even specialize in sporting injuries.

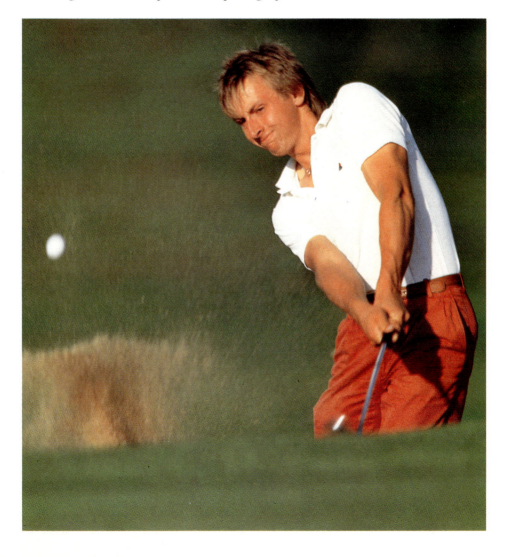

The increased use of typewriters, word processors and VDUs has lead to a corresponding increase in wrist problems among their operators, caused by repetitive stress on these joints. Again, the use of soft-tissue techniques, mobilization and manipulation can help to relieve them.

Chiropractors are also called on to treat problems of the joints in the hands, feet, toes and fingers.

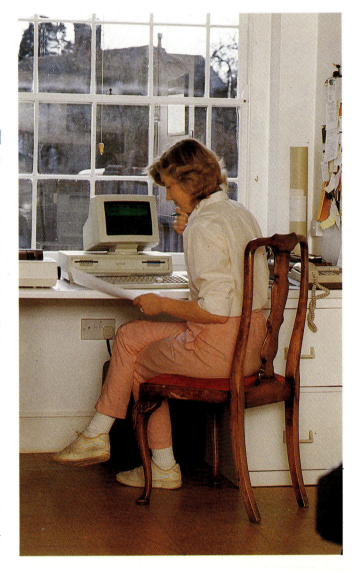

Typewriters, word processors and VDUs frequently cause problems with the neck, shoulders and wrist as well as headaches.

Do's and Dont's at the VDU.

Do...
- sit in a good chair
- use adequate back support
- use a desk of a good height
- take breaks occasionally to rest eyes, neck and shoulders
- stand up and walk around at least once an hour
- loosen neck and shoulders while sitting
- relax wrists while typing

Don't...
- slouch
- sit in a bad chair
- use a low desk or table
- sit for too long at a time
- tense your neck, shoulders or wrist
- use a manual typewriter if possible

Other disorders

A chiropractor also treats, on occasion, problems not directly related to the spine or other joints, but which he knows can sometimes respond to spinal manipulation. Typical examples include asthma, for which the upper back and neck are treated; indigestion, for which the upper back is treated; menstrual pains and bowel problems, which also respond to treatment of the low back; and dizziness (vertigo), deafness and ringing in the ears (tinnitus), for which the neck is usually treated. Chiropractic is not a 'cure-all' for these types of conditions, but effective help can frequently be given.

Backs young and old

As mentioned previously, it is not only people who are middle-aged, overweight and unfit who suffer with back problems. Anyone, of any age, can develop such a condition. It is just that the type of problem tends to vary at different ages. A chiropractor's patients range from the newborn to ninety-year-old grandmothers – back trouble is no respecter of age. On the other hand, a seventy- or eighty-year-old grandmother may well be fitter than her teenage grandson!

Babies and children

Surely, you may say, a newborn baby cannot have a spinal problem – it is too young and its spine is not yet properly formed. This may be so, but being born can in some cases put a great strain on the baby's spine, especially the neck. The baby is not able to tell you it hurts, but its displeasure is usually exhibited as continual crying or bouts of colic.

Chiropractic treatment can sometimes alter a baby's demeanour miraculously. If left unchecked, some spinal problems can exhibit themselves in symptoms such as hyperactivity and bed-wetting as the child gets older. Not all of such symptoms are caused entirely by spinal problems, of course, but it is sensible to have the child or baby checked over. A chiropractor uses special gentle manipulation techniques when treating a baby or child, and adapts them to suit each individual case.

More and more schoolchildren and teenagers now seem to be suffering from types of spinal complaints. There are various reasons for this – bad posture, bad seating at school and at home, desks that are too low (resulting in a bad sitting posture) and lack of exercise are a few. If these problems are not identified and corrected when the children are young, they can

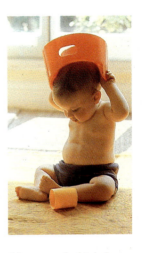

Many people think that a baby's spine is so flexible that it will automatically recover from a fall, accident or even a traumatic birth. This is not always the case. Often these minor traumas will build up over time and cause a spinal problem. Babies and young children don't always feel or show pain in the same way as adults, so the symptoms of the problem may present themselves as colic, crying or sleeplessness, instead.

easily develop into chronic back disorders later in life.

Regular checks for scoliosis should be carried out when children are still at school. Scoliosis is an alteration to the normal straight spine when viewed from the back. It may take up a C-shaped or S-shaped lateral curve. Diagnosis and correction while the child is young can prevent further problems later on. Very often simple exercises can help to stop scoliosis before it develops fully. Only severe cases would require surgery.

Chiropractors usually enjoy treating children because their conditions can be very challenging, and results often come quicker than when treating an older person. Children also tend

Schoolchildren often suffer with back problems due to lack of exercise and badly designed desks and chairs which encourage them to slouch.

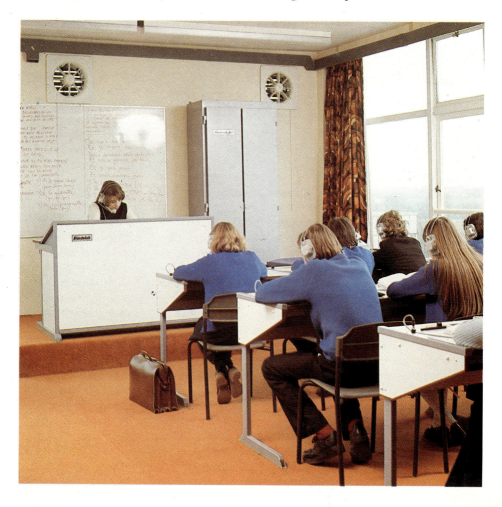

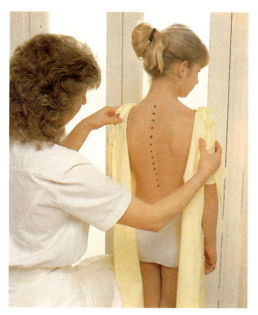 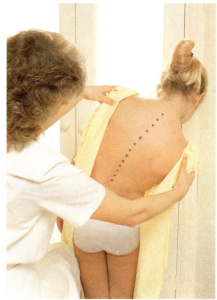

to feel pain in a different way to adults, and to describe it differently as well. It is usually necessary to treat the whole of the spine, because the growing spine continually alters and changes and localized anomalies can have far-reaching effects. An early introduction to back-pain prevention is advisable for all school-aged children, although sadly it is all too commonly neglected.

Older people
At the other end of the human time scale, a great many elderly people are successfully treated using chiropractic therapy. Once somebody is over sixty years old, most aches and pains are put down to age – but with muscle and joint problems in particular this is not necessarily the case. Arthritis and rheumatism may well be present, but need not always cause pain. Pain can arise because of other factors, such as alteration to normal spinal function and tension in the muscles and soft tissues. Great relief can be obtained by treating these problems. As with children, the chiropractor can specially adapt her techniques for treating the elderly, who require a gentler type of therapy than do younger adults. So age, young or old, should not deter anyone from seeing a chiropractor for help or advice as treatment will be modified to suit.

Scoliosis check up in children. Signs of scoliosis (spinal curvature) can develop early in life and all children should be checked regularly for such signs. When caught early, most scoliosis can be halted and helped with chiropractic treatment. Some severe cases however, will still need surgery.

Pregnant women

Pregnancy should be a time of great happiness and good health. But this is not always so for every woman and some pregnant mothers suffer dreadfully with back problems. Ideally, if she wishes to become pregnant, a woman should sort out any back problems first. However, if a back problem does crop up during pregnancy, a chiropractor can still help – the special treatment tables are well adapted to dealing with extra-large abdomens. Indeed many pregnant women are treated by chiropractors right up until a day or two before giving birth.

The enlarging abdomen puts a great strain on the low back area, which can lead to muscular strain as well as joint fixations. In exceptional cases, the baby may actually lie on the

Mothers frequently suffer with back pain as a result of lifting and carrying their growing toddlers. Standing with the child balanced on one or other hip also encourages back problems and should definitely be avoided during pregnancy.

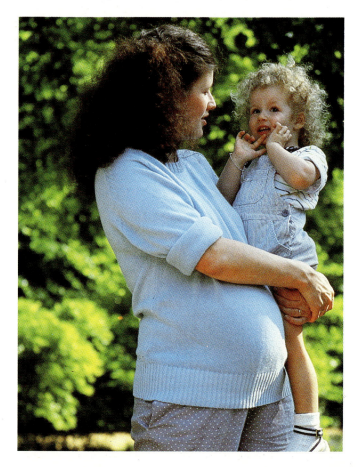

SPORTING INJURIES THAT CHIROPRACTIC CAN HELP		
Athletics Low back pain · Hamstring injuries Hip, knee and ankle problems	**Golf** 'Golfer's' elbow · Low back pain	**Skiing** Knee and cartilage problems
Bodybuilding Low back injuries Shoulder and neck injuries	**Horseriding** Neck problems · Low back problems	**Squash** Low back pain · Disc problems Knee and cartilage problems
Football Groin strains · Hamstring problems Low back pain	**Rugby** Neck problems · Low back pain **Running** Hip, knee and ankle problems Hamstring injuries	**Tennis** Neck, shoulder and arm pain Low back pain · 'tennis' elbow

sciatic nerve, but if this occurs chiropractic treatment cannot help – the mother has to wait until the baby moves.

Back problems can also occur after a difficult birth. The low back may suffer from strain and weakness caused by changes in the pelvis when it expands to let the baby through the birth canal. The back can also be strained when lifting and carrying the baby. Some mothers also suffer from pain in the upper back region because of enlarged breasts, which can put extra stress on the back. By feeding the baby little and often, such strain can be reduced.

Sporting injuries

A group of people who frequently suffer injuries to the back, muscles and joints are those who indulge in sports, both amateur and professional. In professionals, the problem is often aggravated by the fact that they are pushing their body to the limit and seldom have time to rest and recover properly from an injury before the next training session or competition.

Virtually every sport has its characteristic injuries. Most respond extremely well to chiropractic treatment (such as the knee and elbow injuries described earlier). And the sooner treatment is sought, the quicker the problem is solved.

Thus it can be seen that anyone, of any age, can suffer with a back, muscle or joint-related disorder. Chiropractic therapy is well suited to treat such problems, using techniques that can be adapted according to the age, sex, and build of the patient.

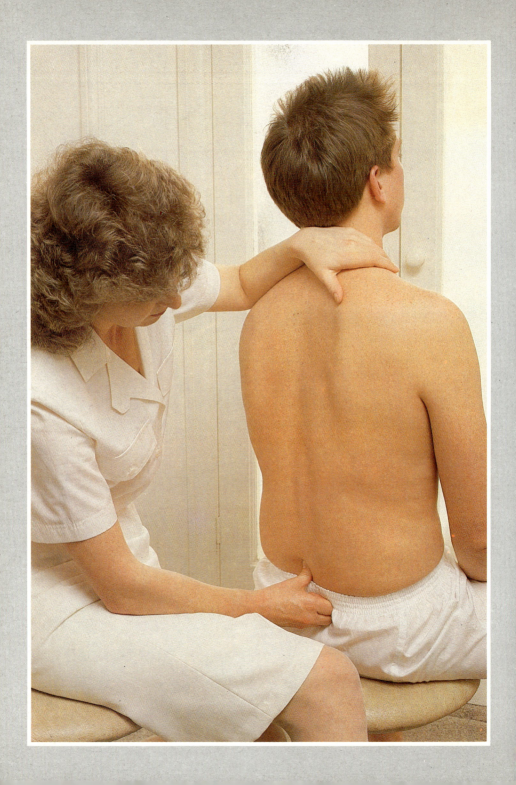

3

CHIROPRACTIC
IN CONTEXT

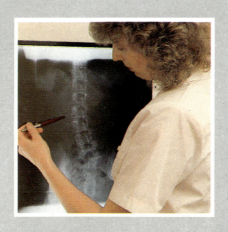

The orthodox medical profession is gradually developing a respect for chiropractors and the forms of treatment they offer. On their side, chiropractors see their profession as being allied to rather than opposed to orthodox medicine. Unlike therapies such as acupuncture, homeopathy and medical herbalism, in which the systems of treatment could be used as a complete alternative to orthodox medicine, chiropractic is seen by most of its practitioners as being complementary.

Many doctors and specialists now refer patients to chiropractors for treatment of their musculoskeletal problems. Correspondingly, chiropractors are trained to refer those conditions not amenable to chiropractic treatment to the appropriate expert. Some orthodox specialists even work closely with chiropractors because they find this a benefit to the patient's condition as a whole. Co-operation in research work is also increasing. This growing association between chiropractic and establishment medical care is a most welcome change from the situation of mutual suspicion that prevailed some years ago.

Chiropractors throughout the world regard themselves as primary health care practitioners. This means that it is possible to consult a chiropractor in the first instance without needing to be referred by your family doctor. A patient can feel confident that the chiropractor is qualified within her scope of practice, and can readily recognize conditions for which referral to the appropriate specialist is necessary.

The advantages of chiropractic

The results of clinical research have shown that manual therapy as administered by qualified chiropractors is safe and effective in the relief of pain that is of a biomechanical origin. Millions of spinal manipulations are carried out each year by chiropractors, and the safety record is extremely good. In fact, because of the physical demands made of the therapist, it is more likely that the chiropractor will be injured while giving the spinal adjustment than that the patient will be injured receiving it.

The education and practical training of a qualified chiropractor are such that she is able to determine whether there are any contra-indications – that is, signs that a form of treatment is inappropriate – to spinal manipulation, or whether the patient should be receiving medical as well as chiropractic care. Chiropractors are taught diagnostic skills that enable them to tell the significance of the different types of symptoms that a patient may exhibit. For instance, they are trained specifically to diagnose the origins and causes of various kinds of pain. Doing this is not always straightforward, because some disorders present symptoms that may initially seem confusing. For example, early symptoms of some kidney or gynaecological disorders actually mimic a low back pain. In such cases, a chiropractor can identify the cause, and then refer the patient to a doctor for confirmation of the diagnosis.

Studies in North America, Europe and Australia show that the great majority of patients visit a chiropractor for disorders related directly to muscles or joints, for which chiropractic treatment is particularly effective. Chiropractic has also been shown to have a success rate of nearly 90 per cent in the treatment of low back and leg pain that is of a biomechanical origin. Furthermore, this type of treatment is generally considered to be remarkably cost-effective.

The patient's case history, combined with examination procedures and the study of X-rays, helps to lead the chiropractor to a diagnosis and a corresponding treatment regime that is best suited to each case on an individual basis. It is usually said that if a pain is relieved by movement and heat, the patient will benefit from manipulation. If, however, the pain is aggravated by movement, then inflammation and acute injury are likely to be present and these should be treated with rest and the application of ice-packs. In either case, the chiropractor is capable of advising the patient and modifying treatment techniques to suit the individual problem.

Associated therapies

As a primary health care practitioner, a chiropractor inevitably encounters conditions for which the normal skills of chiropractic are either inappropriate or inadequate. In such circumstances the chiropractor's diagnostic skills ensure that referral to the correct specialist is done swiftly and effectively. The specialists to which chiropractic is most closely related – and to whom patients are most commonly referred – include physiotherapists, orthopaedists, neurologists and rheumatologists, all of whom are concerned with musculoskeletal problems in general.

One important factor in the referral process is that specialists in all of these fields normally have direct access to modern hospital equipment and analytical facilities, which enable them to carry out extensive testing and examination of the patient in order to clarify the problem and diagnose the complaint. Such

Casenote Ms S suffered with an acute neck pain and some referred pain in the left arm following a car accident in which she sustained a whiplash neck injury. She had already received physiotherapy treatment, which had not helped her condition. As Ms S had already had about six weeks off work with the problem, her medical practitioner decided to refer her to a chiropractor for treatment. She was back at work after a couple of chiropractic treatments and the pain and discomfort were soon resolved.

facilities are usually not available to the chiropractor, and so the need for further investigation is one of the commonest reasons for a patient being referred. Although most musculoskeletal conditions can be treated to some extent by a chiropractor, the following summaries indicate the areas in which treatment by other specialists may be more appropriate.

Physiotherapy Physiotherapists treat musculoskeletal conditions using a variety of treatment regimes, techniques and therapeutic equipment combined with massage, exercise, mobilization and even, on occasion, manipulation. Perhaps most importantly, however, physiotherapists specialize in the physical rehabilitation of patients – for example, as part of the recovery process from an accident, surgery, serious or

Chiropractors and physiotherapists carry out quite different treatment regimes. Chiropractors specialize in treating muscle and joint problems using manipulation, whereas physiotherapists offer a variety of different regimes and concentrate on rehabilitation, which is an area of therapy in which chiropractors are not so involved.

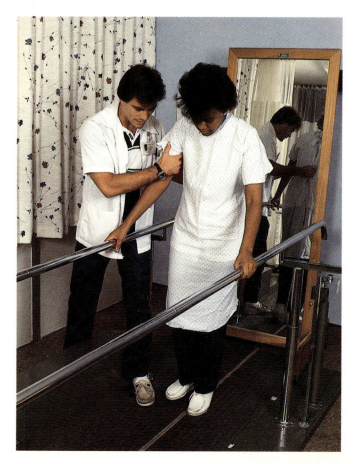

prolonged illness, heart attacks and periods of enforced muscle disuse, which occur when a person is confined to bed or a wheelchair. A chiropractor would not infringe on these areas, although in some cases chiropractors and physiotherapists work side by side for the benefit of the patient. It is certainly the view of chiropractors that this sort of co-operation should be encouraged.

Other specialists A chiropractor is frequently consulted about arthritic conditions, typically those affecting the hips or knees, which should be referred to an orthopaedic surgeon, perhaps for a replacement joint. Other orthopaedic problems such as sprains or fractures may need immobilization in a plaster cast, and problems with the patellar cartilage of the knee may require surgery. Chiropractors are also likely to be consulted by patients with conditions such as a severe spinal prolapse (slipped disc), narrowing of the spinal canal or severe spinal instability, all of which may require the intervention of an orthopaedic surgeon.

Conditions of this type may be associated with nerve damage and, if so, the expertise of a neurologist is needed to make a differential diagnosis and prescribe the appropriate treatment. In certain cases, a neurosurgeon may even be called upon.

A chiropractor is also frequently faced with patients suffering from rheumatological complaints, such as rheumatoid arthritis, and treatment of these requires the intervention of a rheumatologist.

Some conditions that are not ideally suited to chiropractic treatment may not necessarily be referred to an orthodox specialist. In many cases the patient may have already consulted his or her family doctor, who was unable to help them. In such cases, an alternative form of therapy may well be required and the chiropractor might refer the patient to an acupuncturist, homeopath or medical herbalist for treatment.

The aim of the chiropractor is always to ensure that the patient receives the most appropriate treatment in the shortest possible time. To this end, it is essential that there is as much access and inter-referral as possible between chiropractors and the various medical specialists. Unfortunately, many health professionals still feel a suspicion of chiropractors, despite the fact that chiropractors are well aware of the specialized nature of their field and are careful to limit the scope of their practice to conditions of musculoskeletal origin.

Casenote Mrs B was suffering from a dull, achy low back pain which was fairly constant although relieved by heat and rest. Examination by the chiropractor did not reveal any spinal problems that could account for this discomfort. However, questioning did reveal that Mrs B was having lower abdominal pain and some changes in the frequency and heaviness of her menstrual periods. As it was likely that the back pain was the result of a gynaecological problem, Mrs B was referred to the appropriate specialist.

Disorders chiropractic cannot treat

Although chiropractic is an excellent form of therapy for musculoskeletal conditions, there are several types of disorders for which it is inappropriate, even though at first sight this might not seem to be the case. A chiropractor does have some other treatment techniques apart from manipulation, but where these too are not suitable, the patient is normally referred elsewhere.

The first of these groups of disorders affects the bones and joints. It includes conditions such as acute inflammatory arthritis, rheumatoid arthritis, ankylosing spondilitis in the acute and inflamed stages, cervical spondilitis accompanied by circulatory problems in the neck, ruptured ligaments, dislocations and the initial stages of acute injury. This first group also includes conditions such as bone thinning (osteoporosis), bone

As there are certain conditions which should not be treated by manipulation, it is very important that the chiropractor is able to distinguish diagnostically between the conditions he can treat and those he cannot. The rigorous training which the chiropractor undergoes makes her ideally suited to cope with such diagnostic problems. Here the chiropractor is carrying out part of this examination procedure.

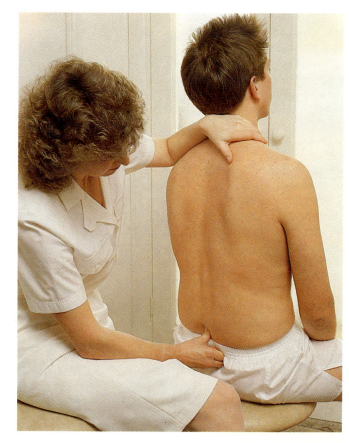

fractures and the presence of bone infection or cancer. None of these conditions should be treated by direct spinal adjustment therapy. On the other hand, people suffering from back pain caused by hypermobile joints (that move too freely) would probably benefit from modified chiropractic treatment.

In summary, manual therapy to the spine is usually contra-indicated when a bone or joint disease is present, or in the absence of any joint dysfunction. However, a chiropractor can use soft-tissue manipulative techniques to help ease muscle spasm in the areas affected or treat the regions above or below the trouble spot, in order to relieve pain.

The second group is made up of circulatory disorders. If the patient suffers from problems with the arteries, such as bulges in the arterial wall (aneurysm), blocked arteries (atherosclerosis), or vertebral artery disease, then manipulation to the neck

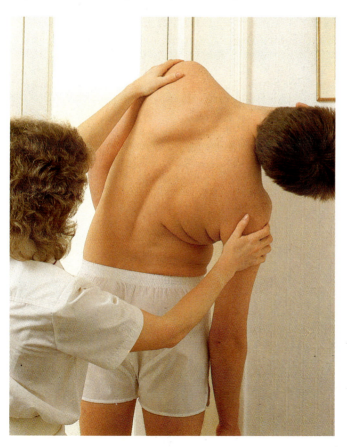

Casenote Mr G was suffering with an extremely acute and severe low back pain, referred pain and pins and needles in the back of the right leg and foot. Examination revealed that the most likely cause of the problem was disc prolapse. Further questioning revealed the recent onset of bladder incontinence. As bladder incontinence can be the result of nerve pressure from the disc, Mr G was immediately referred to a specialist who decided to operate within 24 hours.

This is a typical problem where chiropractic manipulation would not have been suitable.

and low back may be contra-indicated.

The third category includes patients suffering from disc problems in the low back. Manipulation will not benefit the conditions if the problem is accompanied by serious neurological changes, such as loss of bladder control. In these cases, referral to a surgeon is imperative.

The fourth and last group consists of patients with psychological problems. Some patients are so frightened of manipulation, or of the discomfort it might involve, that they automatically tense and resist the treatment. The chiropractor tries to talk the patient through his or her fear, explaining the procedures, but does not always succeed. In such cases an alternative treatment regime is recommended.

Chiropractic and osteopathy

Both chiropractic and osteopathy were founded in the nineteenth century, in the United States, by men of determination and vision who were dissatisfied by the health care that was generally available at the time. Chiropractic was founded in 1895 in Iowa, by Daniel David Palmer. Osteopathy was founded nearly 20 years earlier (in 1874) by Dr Andrew Taylor Still, a country doctor in neighbouring Missouri.

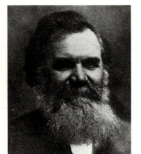

Daniel David Palmer 1845-1913.

Origins Still was emotionally shattered when three of his children died from meningitis. His distress was compounded because he felt frustrated by his inability to do anything to prevent their deaths. The science of medicine at that time proved inadequate to save their lives and, from his disillusionment with orthodox practice, he turned his mind to considering fundamental questions of health and disease.

His studies led him to the conclusion that the body is a vital machine with an anatomical structure and physiological functions. If the body is structurally normal, it will be healthy. Still claimed that structural distortions of the body interfere with the circulation of blood, which in turn lead to ill-health and disease. By correcting structural problems through mechanical methods, which Still developed as the basis of osteopathy, the circulation can be restored and the body returned to health.

Unfortunately, Still had difficulty in persuading his colleagues in the medical profession of the efficiency of his form of treatment and he was forced to move on from one place to another until he finally settled in Kirksville, Missouri. It was there in 1892 that he founded the first school of osteopathy to teach his theories and techniques to others.

Palmer shared Still's view that the body's physical structure governs its function, but thought that it was interference with the nervous system through structural distortion that causes functional disease. Palmer also developed a mechanical system to correct these functional problems. In 1896, he opened the first school of chiropractic, called Dr Palmer's School and Cure, in Davenport, Iowa. This was later to become the Palmer Institute and Chiropractic Infirmary.

Early development Not surprisingly, during the early development of the two professions Palmer was accused of having stolen ideas from Still. Although the truth will probably never be known for certain, it is a fact that Kirksville, Missouri, was only one day's journey from Davenport, Iowa, and Palmer did visit Kirksville. It is questionable if he took anything from Still's concepts, but they did meet in the 1890s.

Osteopathy developed more rapidly than chiropractic at first and at the turn of the century there were 1,136 osteopaths in the United States, but fewer than 100 chiropractors. By the 1930s, however, although the number of osteopathic physicians had increased to 7,654, they were significantly outnumbered by more than 16,000 chiropractors.

Because the two professions in the United States developed in different directions, the competition between them there has lessened. Osteopathy developed more in the direction of orthodox medicine and, although osteopaths in the United States still practise a certain amount of manipulation, in most states they also prescribe drugs and practise surgery. It is interesting to note that this would be against the beliefs of osteopaths in Britain, unless confronted with a matter of life and death. By contrast, chiropractic in the United States remained an alternative profession, filling the gaps left by the osteopathic manipulators who had turned to more orthodox medical practice.

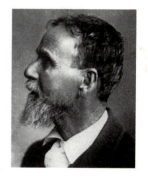

Dr Andrew Taylor Still 1828-1917.

In Britain, the British Osteopathic Association was formed in 1910. Although chiropractors have practised in Britain since the turn of the century, it was not until 1925 that the British Chiropractic Association was formed by a group of 18 chiropractors who had qualified in the United States. At the Sixth Annual Conference of the BCA, the European Chiropractor's Union was formed, with practitioners from Belgium, Denmark, Sweden and Switzerland joining their British colleagues.

This is quite a typical osteopathic technique for stiffness and ache between the shoulder blades. Chiropractors would tend to treat the same problem, but using different manipulative techniques.

Chiropractic and osteopathy today   Chiropractic is now the largest manipulative profession in the world, with practitioners active in most countries. All chiropractors who belong to recognized national associations have the same standard of education and practical training, which means that a chiropractor who qualified in Britain could go to almost any other country and find another chiropractor working in a similar way using similar techniques. This does not occur to the same extent with osteopaths, whose science is considerably more

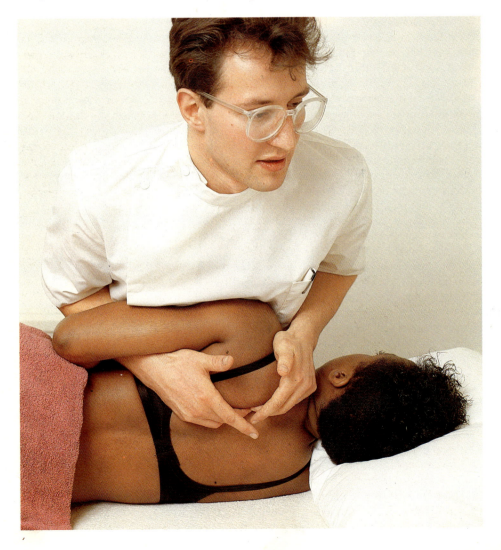

diverse in its principles of practice, and a similar uniformity cannot be found.

Over the decades, both professions have moved away from the early ideas about the circulation or the nervous system ruling the body in such a way that interference with either system causes ill health.

Today, chiropractic and osteopathy both concentrate on the structural and mechanical disorders that occur in the body and can lead to musculoskeletal problems. Nevertheless, osteopaths tend to lay more emphasis on the interrelationship between skeletal structure and organ systems as they effect a patient's general health than most chiropractors do.

Apart from their general differences in approach to illness and its treatment, chiropractors and osteopaths also differ considerably in the practical ways they deal with patients' disorders. A patient who consulted both a chiropractor and an osteopath would notice a number of important differences. The most obvious of these is that chiropractors make greater use of X-ray equipment as an aid to diagnosis. Each specialist also employs quite different treatment regimes.

The chiropractic treatment might typically consist of soft-tissue massage or, in certain cases, the use of an adjunct such as an ultra-sound machine. This may then be followed by specific spinal or joint adjustment to restore normal movement to the structural system, using a high-velocity, low-amplitude movement of the practitioner's hand or hands.

In a comparable situation, an osteopath might use a number of different techniques. These may include soft-tissue massage, although an osteopath's technique for this feels more forceful than the touch of a chiropractor. The osteopath may apply passive articulation techniques which aim to stretch the tissues using different parts of the body as levers. He may also try a high-velocity thrust (HVT) technique to move the joints, but here also the method used and the feel of the osteopath's touch will differ and usually be more forceful than those the patient would encounter at the hands of a chiropractor.

Chiropractic research

One would be forgiven for thinking that chiropractic research is a feature of the present rather than of the past. Interestingly, however, this is not the case. As early as the 1930s, B J Palmer, the son of D D Palmer, who took over his father's fledgling school for chiropractors, was carrying out research in the field, and established a research clinic at the school in 1935. His

Chiropractors and osteopaths treat the same type of muscle and joint related problems, but their manipulative techniques vary greatly. In the USA, osteopaths concentrate more on treatments using drugs and surgery rather than using their manipulative skills.

Chiropractors
Second largest primary health care profession worldwide
● Use specific contact adjustive techniques
● Same educational standards worldwide
● Use X-rays as an aid to diagnosis

Osteopaths
Profession concentrated in UK and USA
● Use more mobilization techniques
● Use more soft-tissue techniques
● Use more lever type adjustive techniques

establishment was so well-equipped and its staff were so competent that it became one of the finest clinics in the American Midwest. Among B J Palmer's triumphs was the instrument he developed in 1935, for reading brain waves and picking up their pathways along the spinal cord. This was a prototype of the EEG (electroencephalograph), with which doctors are so familiar today.

This scientific and investigative approach does not coincide with many popular views of chiropractic, however. Among orthodox practitioners in particular there has long been a delight in telling tales of chiropractic treatment that had gone wrong – by implication because there was no sound scientific basis for the chiropractor's technique. In reply, chiropractors have collected equally dogmatic stories of false diagnosis, inappropriate treatment and over-prescription of drugs by orthodox doctors. Attempts to reinforce these antagonistic views have focused on scorning the system on which the practice is based.

Members of the orthodox medical profession have pointed to what they see as a lack of scientific evidence to explain or prove how chiropractic manipulation actually works. However, such an absence of hard theoretical evidence for techniques and treatments that work in practice is relatively commonplace in other fields of medicine. Many of the health care procedures we take for granted today have never been subjected to randomized controlled trials. And even when a trial suggests that a medical procedure may in fact be useless, despite the evidence of its past success, this verdict often has very little effect – the procedure continues to be used and, illogically, to succeed.

Clinical trials Statistically, the most reliable method of research is a randomized clinical trial, in which patients are randomly assigned to one type of treatment or another. This is also the most expensive type of assessment in terms of both time and finance. The other essential feature of a clinical trial is that it should be carried out 'double-blind'. This means that neither the patient nor the researcher knows what type of treatment is being given – for example, a 'sham' manipulation instead of an actual one. Because of the enormous costs involved in clinical trials, however, it is only in the last ten years that specialists in the fields of physical medicine have been able to begin using them.

At the time of writing, however, there are four controlled

Palmer's first patient D D Palmer's first patient is believed to have been the janitor of his apartment building. This janitor had suffered with deafness for some years after he had heard something go 'crack' in his neck. Palmer worked out that if there was pressure on a nerve, deafness could be the result of a type of referred pain. He then adjusted the janitor's neck and 'miraculously' restored his hearing.

chiropractic trials currently being conducted in the United States, Canada and Britain. Two of these are taking place in the United States. One is concerned with patients with mild chronic low back pain, and compares spinal adjustive therapy with no active treatment. The other compares the chiropractic and orthodox medical management of chronic low back pain. The latter American test is being duplicated in the Canadian trial. In Britain, the trial is comparing chiropractic and hospital out-patient management of patients with a specific type of low back pain of mechanical origin.

Each of these trials has required extensive co-operation between medical and chiropractic professionals, combined with a great deal of financial backing and resources. Nevertheless, it will be ten years from the start of each trial before the results can be correlated.

Other research A less costly form of research involves descriptive studies – looking at how patients respond to a certain treatment. Research of this kind is being undertaken continually throughout the world and is reported regularly in medical journals. Examples include: case control studies, in which patients are studied during and after treatment; observational studies, which are similar to case control studies without the actual involvement of the patients; and case studies, in which only certain individual cases are reported.

The future Everyone agrees that there is a great need for qualified chiropractors who are also qualified researchers, able to initiate and control more research and trials of an internationally recognized nature. A general view at present is that chiropractic research should be directed towards three main areas: the evaluation of chiropractic diagnostic techniques; the evaluation of chiropractic therapy; and the evaluation of basic science studies. Comprehensive analysis of these three areas requires a combination of laboratory, field and clinical study.

As chiropractic colleges increase in size, number and funding and as inter-professional links are forged, increasing collaboration in research will also be necessary. Research is needed not only to compare the effectiveness of different types of treatment on different conditions, but also to understand exactly what is happening to the body on a microscopic level when the spine is manipulated. We must also find out exactly how far-reaching the effects of manipulation are.

The commonest ailments Approximately 90 per cent of general medical practice involves treatment for the common cold, back pain, headache and indigestion. Except for the common cold, treatment is usually by trial and error as it can often be impossible to make an exact diagnosis.

Bed rest Back sufferers are usually given bed rest as the immediate form of treatment and the time they are confined to bed can vary from a few days to a number of weeks.

Evidence now suggests that bed rest may not always be the best aid to recovery because:
- it inhibits healing
- muscle strength is lost by 3 per cent a day
- bones start to lose minerals
- fitness decreases
- psychological distress and depression increase
- rehabilitation is retarded

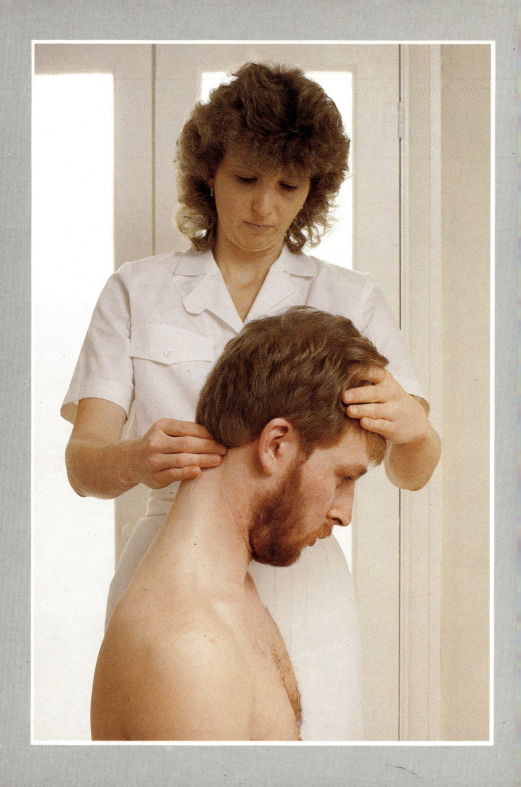

4

HOW
CHIROPRACTIC
WORKS

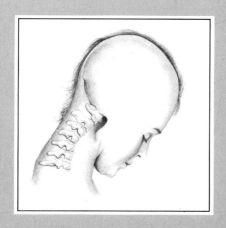

A major element of chiropractic therapy involves adjustment and manipulation of the spine in order to re-establish the normal positions and functions of nerves, which in turn influence other parts of the body. As a technique, spinal manipulation is used therapeutically by practitioners in three major healing professions: chiropractors, osteopaths and medical manipulators.

It is generally understood that manipulation as carried out by medical doctors and physiotherapists involves the forceful, passive movement of a joint beyond its active limit of motion. 'Passive' refers to the patient, who takes no part in the technique other than let it happen. The technique for this procedure involves using parts of the body (such as the arms and legs) as long levers to make the movements. The reasoning behind this technique is that manipulation used on a stiff or painful joint will stop the pain and cure the stiffness. With a bit of luck one treatment may be enough, although usually two or three are required. If the pain is relieved the treatment is a success; if not, another form of therapy is tried.

The practice of chiropractic adjustment is an art which takes many years to perfect. In qualified hands, spinal manipulation is safe, but it is an exact therapy which relies on the precision of the practitioner not only in performing the adjustment itself but also in the placing and positioning of the patient prior to adjustment as shown here.

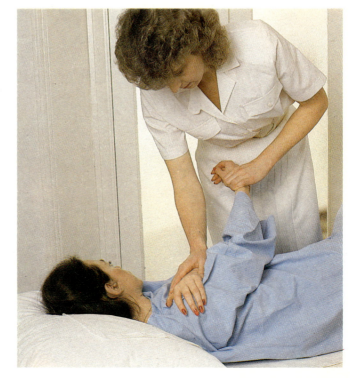

In contrast, spinal manipulation as carried out by a chiropractor or osteopath is aimed at restoring normal joint function and reducing any effects on the body through the nervous or circulatory systems. Chiropractors and osteopaths look for the areas of the spine that are not functioning normally. They then use spinal manipulation to restore normal function and mobility over a period of time, and treatment ceases only when normal movement is restored and the pain and any other symptoms relieved. It is therefore a much more complex system of treatment than simple medical manipulation.

Chiropractic manipulation is frequently also described as adjustment. It involves a short-lever, high-velocity movement with a specific contact on the spine by the therapist's hand or hands using a steady controlled force. Although this may sound complicated, in fact the movements made by a chiropractor are slight but very quick. With this type of manipulative technique, the positioning of the joint to be adjusted is of vital importance so that the adjustment can be

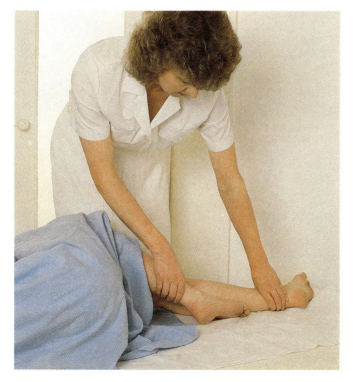

Sometimes the patient is in such pain that any movement will increase it. In such cases the chiropractor will take great care to place the patient very gently in the right position before adjustment or manipulation.

performed with minimum force but maximum precision.

Manipulative techniques of this kind cannot be learned in a few days or weeks, and the internationally accepted standard training for a chiropractor is equivalent to a full-time four-year course. To maintain the skills of spinal adjustment, the chiropractor has to be in regular practice.

Mobilization and manipulation

The differences between the two therapies of mobilization and manipulation of a joint or joints are quite distinct. To appreciate these differences, consider the following movements of your head and neck, which demonstrate what a chiropractor understands by active movement, mobilization and manipulation.

If the therapist asks you to turn your head to one side as far as it will go, you will take it to the end of its active range of movement.

The therapist can then move the head a bit further using her hand, with a slight pressure on the head. This then takes the head to the end of its passive range of movement, and constitutes mobilization.

When adjusting the spine, the chiropractor will take the spinal joints to the limit of their anatomical integrity (as far as they can go before dislocation) and will then apply the quick thrust that will adjust and mobilize the joint or joints.

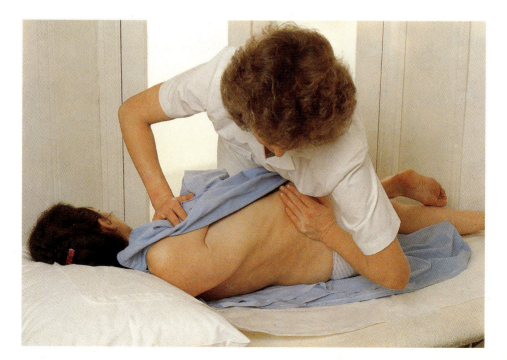

When the end of this passive range of movement is reached, there is an elastic barrier of resistance. If the joint surfaces are forced beyond the elastic barrier, they suddenly move apart and free themselves. This type of movement, frequently accompanied by a cracking noise, constitutes a manipulation.

Many people worry about the cracking noise when the joints move. It is caused by the sudden freeing of gas (carbon dioxide) in the synovial fluid between the joint surfaces, and is similar to the noise one hears when someone cracks his finger joints. The gas bubbles take about thirty minutes to reform, and during that time there is an increase in the size of the joint space while the elastic barrier of resistance is absent. As the synovial gases are re-absorbed, the elastic barrier re-establishes itself. Until this happens, however, the joint can be unstable and it is not usually advisable to re-manipulate it in this condition.

Forcing the joint past this barrier causes physical damage to the joint and joint capsule. A skilled manipulator therefore has to judge the exact positioning required for a joint and the precise amount of force needed to restore joint mobility without damaging it anatomically.

The chiropractor is able to draw on experience of different manipulative techniques to find the one most suited to each individual patient. Here she is adjusting the low back using a different adjustment more suitable in this case.

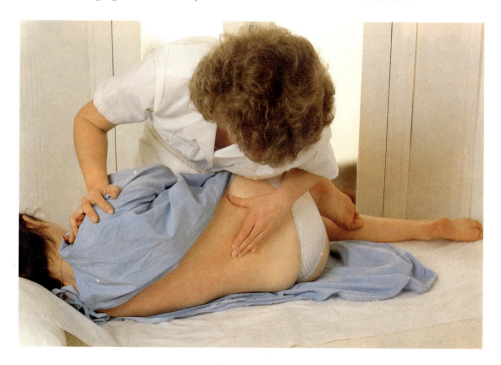

A spinal adjustment as carried out by a chiropractor can be described as the application of a force to a specific, localized area of the body. The force has to be delivered with a controlled depth and magnitude through a specific contact on a particular part of the bone – such as the bony projections called processes on a vertebra. Controlling this adjustment requires considerable skill and practice to ensure the manipulation is delivered with exactly the right amount of speed, force and amplitude. Chiropractors receive lengthy training for this; see chapter 8, Finding and Consulting a Chiropractor.

The aim of chiropractic adjustment

Chiropractic adjustment aims to restore the normal function to the joints being adjusted. This can in turn bring about changes in other parts of the body through the effects of adjustment on the nervous and circulatory systems.

The purpose of the adjustment can therefore be described as the correction of any misalignments of the bones, and the correction of the mobility – or lack of it – between the joint surfaces. At times, the adjustment aims to correct a combination of misalignment and joint dysfunctions at the same time. Loss of normal joint function that continues without correction can eventually produce permanent structural damage, which can then result in a chronic and disabling problem at some time in the future.

The biomechanics of muscle and joint disorders

D D Palmer, the founder of chiropractic, described his philosophy behind chiropractic in the following terms:

'The amount of nerve tension determines health or disease. In health there is normal tension, known as tone, the normal activity, strength and excitability of the various organs and functions as observed in a state of health. The kind of disease depends upon what nerves are too tense or too slack.'

This was a good theory to build on a hundred years ago, but rather overstated the case. We now know that infections, for example, are caused by viruses and bacteria; we know that chiropractic adjustment cannot cure cancer; and we know that heart attacks are not due to spinal nerve tension. The idea that nerves can be too tense or too slack and thereby cause disease is also no longer acceptable.

Casenote Ms A was suffering with pain in the low back, upper back and neck pain as a result of jarring the spine three weeks previously. She first suffered with back pain at the age of thirteen when her medical practitioner discovered spinal scoliosis (sideways curvature of the spine). No treatment had been given. After examination, the chiropractor found that Ms A still had scoliosis with an area of stress at the top of the lower spine and increased vertebral movement and muscle spasm in the area. After four treatments the problem was resolved and Ms A found that she could keep it under control with 3-6 monthly preventive check-ups.

It remains the case that the spinal adjustment D D Palmer gave his janitor Harvey Lillard to cure his deafness did work. This first treatment constituted a simple clinical trial in that it involved a technique (the adjustment) to correct spinal function with a desired clinical outcome – the restoration of hearing. Thus Palmers' initial hypothesis – that adjusting the spine restores spinal function, which in turn then promotes health and reduces disease – had some merit both clinically and scientifically. To convert these theories into terms that can be applied today, however, we must first define clearly what we mean by disease.

Today the chiropractic approach is that of a biomechanic. A chiropractor looks for areas of the spine and joints in which the spinal mechanics are altered, that is to say, where there is either too little or too much movement compared to normal. The chiropractor then seeks to correct the altered mechanics using an adjustment to the spine or other joint in order to restore normal function. Because of the complexities of the body and the interrelationship of the muscular and nervous systems with the skeletal system, correcting any one of these systems inevitably alters the others as well.

This is because disorders of the nerves, muscles and bones (the neuromusculoskeletal system) can be transmitted two ways: in reflexes conducted either from the spine to the internal organs; or from the internal organs on to the spine. These can then manifest themselves in specific related disorders. When one system is not functioning properly it brings about a condition of 'dis-ease' in the others, thus upsetting their normal functions as well. This can result in a variety of symptoms in the system or systems concerned and even in the internal organs. Continued 'dis-ease' in a system can weaken it to such an extent that its general resistance is lowered, thus exposing it to infections which may lead ultimately to real disease.

It is in this way that a chiropractor sees the links between the three systems, and later we shall see how they can be affected by the three major causes of 'dis-ease' – mechanical, chemical and physiological trauma.

Finding a spinal or joint malfunction and simply correcting it is not all there is to chiropractic, however. Detecting such problems is a science, and correcting them is an art. The science of detection involves the patient's case history, orthopaedic, neurological and chiropractic examination, and possibly analysis using X-rays. Then the diagnosis has to be

Casenote Ms Y aged 33 had noticed chest pains around the breastbone two years previously. Exertion, damp and cold aggravated the problem and the pain was relieved with rest. All orthodox examinations were unhelpful.

The chiropractor found an area of tenderness and restriction around the 4th, 5th and 6th upper back vertebrae and ribs. Treatment of the spine soon resolved the pain and after five treatments, Ms Y was fully recovered.

There are different adjustive techniques for treating each part of the spine. This is because of the different configurations, build and shape of the various parts of the spine, each requiring a particular amount of force and line of drive in the application of the adjustment. This is one method of adjusting the middle of the upper back using a technique known as 'diversified'.

made. And after that the chiropractor has to use her art in spinal or joint manipulation to bring about changes in the neuromuscular and skeletal systems to free the patient from his or her clinical problem – be it pain, discomfort, headache or migraine. Thus chiropractic can be described as a scientific discipline more akin to medicine and engineering than to physics.

Today's disturbed joint function creates stress that produces tomorrow's permanent structural damage. Skilled spinal adjustment can correct not only local problems, but can also influence body function and many diseased states through direct, indirect or reflex nerve mechanisms. And however it works, the ultimate aim of chiropractic is the promotion of good health.

How is adjustment achieved?

There are some 36 different types of chiropractic adjustment techniques. The ones most commonly used consist of either a 'dynamic' or a high-velocity thrust adjustment, or a 'recoil' adjustment.

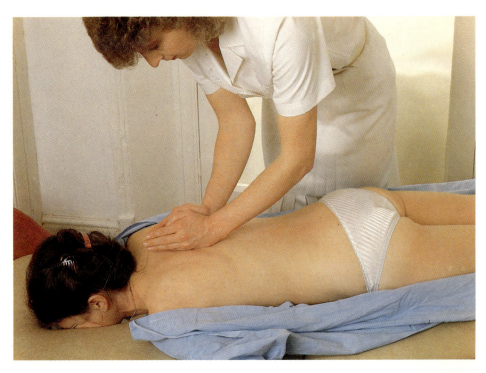

In a recoil adjustment, the patient usually lies in a neutral and relaxed position, often face down on the treatment table. The chiropractor makes contact with the edge of her palm on a specific joint to be adjusted and removes any slack from the skin so that a tight contact is obtained. She gives a very fast thrust to the joint through the contact of her hand on the surface of the skin. This thrust has a high speed, but a low amplitude or depth in order to avoid any damage to the structures in the area.

With the dynamic or high–velocity thrust adjustment, the part of the body being adjusted has to be positioned so that the joint is at the limit of its active range of motion. For the low back, this requires the patient to lie on one side with the upper body twisted in the opposite direction to the pelvis, to introduce an element of rotation and lateral flexion to the spine. This in turn brings the spinal joints to the limit of their active range of movement. By causing a counter–rotation on the spine, achieved by varying the extent to which the hips and knees are bent, a point of tension can be obtained at which the chiropractor makes a specific contact with her hand on the area

Headaches and migraine are frequently associated with an underlying neck problem. Treatment of the neck problem can often help rid the patient of the headache, even if it has been extremely long-standing.

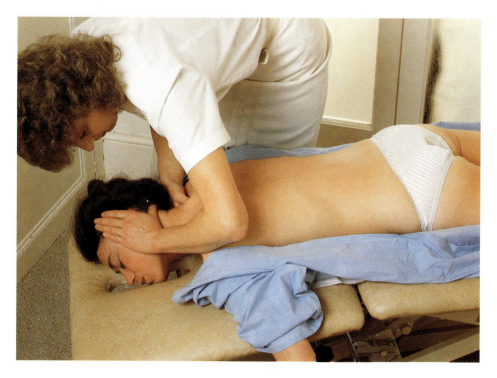

to be adjusted. She then carefully turns the patient's body so that the joint is taken through its range of movement to the elastic barrier of resistance. The chiropractor applies a small thrust, again of high speed but short amplitude. This thrust is given in a specific direction in order to restore normal spinal and joint mechanics, function and integrity. It may be necessary to repeat this action at more than one level in the lumbar spine and first on one side and then the other.

When adjusting the neck, it is positioned so that it is at the end of its passive range of movement. The chiropractor makes contact with the part of the neck to be adjusted, using the edge of her hand or forefinger. Again taking out any slack in the tissue in the neck, she applies a very quick movement with low amplitude. This affects the joint area concerned, again taking it through the elastic barrier of resistance.

Joint fixation

So far we have dealt with the basis of chiropractic adjustment and how the adjustment is achieved. But why does this need to be done in the first place? A fuller description of the biomechanics of spinal and joint function will help to explain the reasoning behind the use of such adjustment or manipulation.

The chiropractor is looking for, and then treating, alterations to the normal function (the dynamics) of the joints. Not only may the dynamics of a particular joint be affected, but also its anatomical and physiological relationships with other parts of the body. The chiropractor frequently calls such alteration a 'fixation'. This term includes any change in the normal function of the particular joint concerned, its related bone, muscular, soft-tissue and nerve function and any changes that occur in the nerve and muscle activity, as well as any effect on nearby vessels – all as a consequence of the joint malfunction.

Other authors and practitioners have described a fixation as a subluxation, a manipulatable lesion, a vertebral lesion or a spinal dysarthria, but for simplicity we shall use the term fixation when discussing alterations to spinal biomechanics in this way.

Various authorities also have different ways of classifying the types of joint or spinal fixations that can occur – it is not normally the case that the joint merely fixes or locks and stops moving. Restriction can occur in a number of different ways. Nor does the effect occur only in the joint itself, but influences

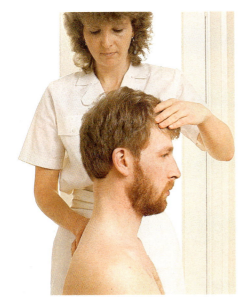 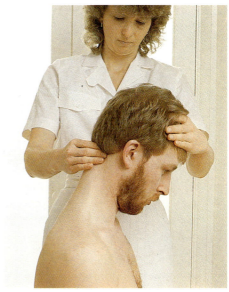

Before adjusting the neck, the chiropractor will examine the dynamics of spinal movement, from the neutral (above), and forward bending positions (above right and right) as well as in backward extension and rotation. In this way areas of altered spinal mobility can be detected. Here the chiropractor is examining the different degrees of forward bending.

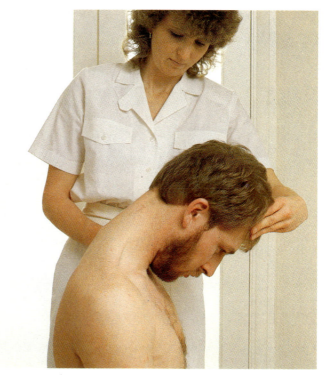

DIFFERENT TYPES OF SPINAL MOVEMENT

normal

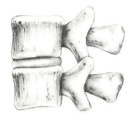

forward bending

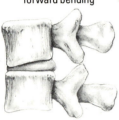

extension

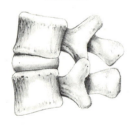

sideways bending

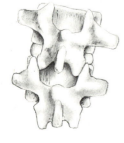

other tissues around and attached to it. The effect can even extend farther afield, because the muscular, nervous and vascular systems can also be involved. When we describe such changes in terms of biomechanics, we include not only a joint but all other associated structures as well – what is termed a motor unit.

The simplest type of fixation occurs when the motor unit is unable to move from its normal resting position, and remains fixed in normal joint alignment. Another type occurs when the joint is unable to move properly through its normal range of movement and is fixed partly in and partly out of alignment. A third type of fixation occurs when the motor unit is unable to return to its normal resting position, and remains fixed outside normal joint alignment.

The situation is further complicated because there are many different causes for joint and motor unit fixations. They can be sub-divided into: static motor unit fixations, kinetic motor unit fixations and structural alterations.

Static motor unit fixations occur when a joint is fixed in one of the following positions: flexion, extension, lateral flexion or rotation.

Flexion fixation occurs when the front of the vertebral bodies come closer together (or approximate) and the back of them separate.

Extension fixation occurs when the front of the vertebral bodies separate and the back of them come together.

Lateral flexion fixation occurs when the vertebral bodies and facets on the side of flexion come together and those on the other side separate.

Rotational fixation occurs when the vertebral bodies rotate to one side, causing tension of the joints on the other side of them.

The various fixations can be further qualified depending on whether one vertebra moves forwards (anterolisthesis), backwards (retrolisthesis) or sideways (laterolisthesis) in relation to the one below it. Another type of static fixation occurs when there is an increase or a reduction in the amount of space between the vertebral bodies. Lastly, narrowing of the intervertebral space – called a foramen – can occur as a result of a mixture of these static types of fixation.

All of these types of changes show up on an ordinary X-ray. Then the therapist, using the keen sense of palpation in her fingertips, is able to detect the fixation by feeling for areas of reduced mobility in the spine and joints. As a result, she can correct it using the joint adjustment or manipulation particularly suited to the type of fixation involved.

Kinetic motor unit fixations involve some sort of fixation of the motor unit that reduces its mobility (hypomobility). To compensate for the loss of mobility, other units in the area move more freely than they should – in other words, they become hypermobile.

Sometimes a hypermobile unit occurs without any associated hypomobility – typical in a professional gymnast, for example. This can cause excessive injury and strain at both microscopic and macroscopic levels. The changes occur at the intervertebral discs, in the associated ligaments and soft tissues,

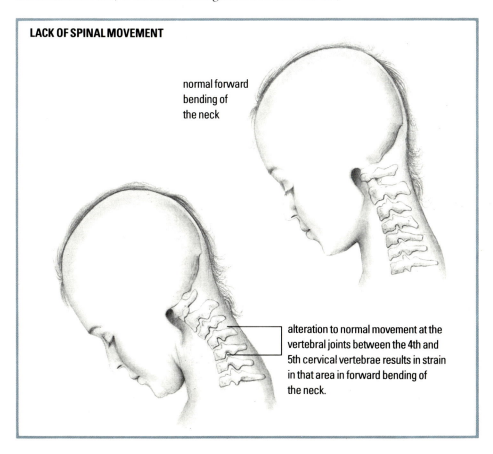

LACK OF SPINAL MOVEMENT

normal forward bending of the neck

alteration to normal movement at the vertebral joints between the 4th and 5th cervical vertebrae results in strain in that area in forward bending of the neck.

and in the spinal muscles. There can also be damage and irritation to the nerve tissue in the spinal canal and intervertebral spaces. Eventually there is excessive wear on the facet joints as well, all leading to early degeneration in the spine.

Another type of kinetic problem occurs when the vertebrae move 'out of synchronization' with each other. For example, when the neck is bent, one of its vertebrae may not flex, and thus moves out of time with the other vertebrae. This type of aberrant movement is usually caused by an injury.

Structural alterations can also induce vertebral fixations because any alteration from the normal design of the spine puts increased stress on other areas, causing them to lock or fix and show signs of strain. A typical example occurs when there is an alteration to the normal spinal curve, such as an increase or decrease in the cervical lordosis (forward curve), an increase or decrease in the thoracic kyphosis (backward curve) or an increase or decrease in the lumbar lordosis. Another example involves scoliosis (a sideways curve in the spine). It can take the form of either a C-shaped or S-shaped curvature that affects part or all of the spine and results in regions of increased stress and altered spinal movement. Bad posture may also lead to an altered spinal structure. Congenital changes to the shape of the vertebrae can lead to asymmetry, which in turn leads to structural alterations and stress areas.

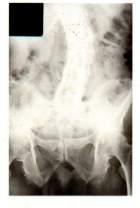

X-rays are an important diagnostic aid to the chiropractor as they often reveal conditions of the spine which are not apparent from an external examination. This x-ray shows a person suffering from ankylosing spondylitis which is a rheumatic disease for which manipulation would not be suitable.

Exercise is good for you, but overuse of a joint, as can happen to gymnasts, can lead to as many problems as not exercising.

Causes of pain

We have seen that there are many ways in which the normal biomechanics of the spine can be altered, but how do these alterations end up producing what we feel as pain and discomfort?

The fixation of a motor unit affects not only the joint itself but also the joint capsule, intervertebral disc, intervertebral ligaments and the attached muscles and tendons.

There may also be neurological effects because of the proximity of the spinal cord and spinal nerves, and because of proprioceptive nerve endings in the structures concerned. These proprioceptive nerve endings sense the positions of the joints and continually relay the information up and down the spinal cord to and from the brain. This barrage of nerve impulses usually only makes matters worse, because the muscular contraction that originally brought on the vertebral fixation is often reinforced. This leads to and perpetuates both

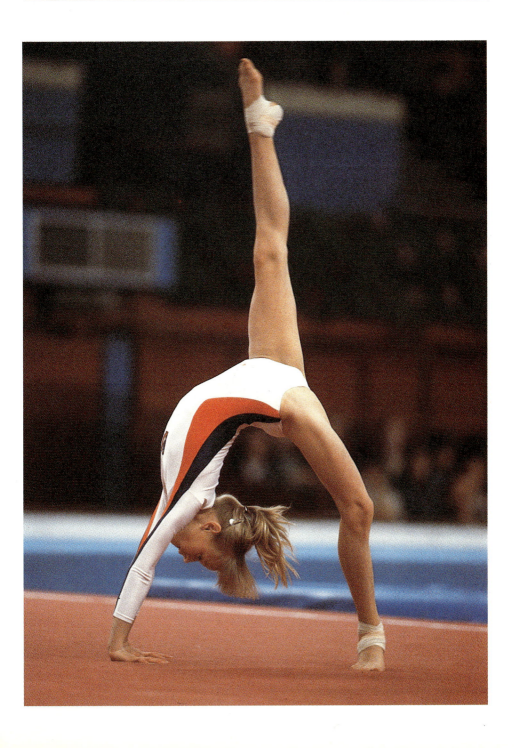

the fixation and any associated conditions.

Associated with a joint fixation there are usually soft-tissue (muscular and ligamentous) changes overlying the affected area. These can be in the form of inflammation, irritation, swelling and even degenerative changes, weakness and loss of tone in the soft tissue itself.

More important, however, are any neurological changes that may occur, because their effects can be more far reaching. Because of the numerous alterations to tissues involved with a joint fixation in the spine, the intervertebral space can become narrowed where the spinal nerve leaves it (usually with a

THE CAUSES OF BACK ACHE

Many things can cause back pain, not all of them obvious as you can see in the chart below. In order to treat sufferers correctly and successfully, the chiropractor has to ask questions about their job, mental state, personal history, hobbies and habits – even what kind of car they drive, as any one of these things could be a primary or contributory cause of the problem.

Mechanical	Chemical	Psychological
Car accidents	Nutritional deficiencies	Stress
Falls		Tension
Lifting	Smoking Infections	Overwork
Bending		Boredom
Bad posture	Excessive heat and cold	Worry
Bad chairs	Electric shock	Marital problems
Soft beds	Foreign bodies in the tissues	Interrelationship problems
Saggy sofas		
Low desks	Bad food combinations	Work dissatisfaction
Car seats	allergies	
Overweight		

compensatory widening elsewhere). The narrowing irritates the nerves, and widening stretches them.

These and any other neurological changes are, in fact, extremely complicated at the microscopic level. Eventually, if left unchecked, they result in pain, and only then does the patient know that a problem has arisen. In certain cases the sensory nerve endings in the musculoskeletal tissues can confuse the issue, because they can influence both the tissues themselves and the internal organs supplied by a particular nerve or group of nerves. As a result, the changes can manifest themselves as pain in the nerves, in the tissues or even in an internal organ (for example, in the stomach, causing indigestion).

When a chiropractor examines the spine and finds a vertebral fixation, she is nearly always also able to detect changes in the soft tissues overlying the area. This is because the fixation affects the flow of blood and lymph in nearby vessels, making it sluggish, which in turn may be accompanied by such other tissue changes as swelling (oedema), lack of oxygen, and the build up of toxins. This then leads to a disturbance in the normal exchange of nutrients and waste products through the circulatory and lymphatic systems. The function of the muscles will be affected, as will the nerves. Thus the overall manifestation of the group of problems is pain and discomfort, perhaps with pins and needles or numbness.

The causes of joint fixations

We have considered the biomechanics and changes to nerves and tissues involved in a joint fixation. But what, in the first instance, actually causes it?

It is generally agreed that there are three possible causes of joint fixations: mechanical irritants, chemical irritants and psychological trauma.

Mechanical irritants   These form a category that includes the greatest number of different causes of joint fixation.

One of the most common is injury (trauma) resulting from a fall or other accident. Falls jar the spine and can initiate a joint fixation. Car accidents resulting in a whiplash injury to the neck can often cause an immediate problem, with damage not only to the joints but also to the overlying soft tissues. Another common category of injuries occur at work, particularly those caused by lifting heavy objects or repeatedly lifting things awkwardly.

Casenote Mr W suffered with pain in the neck, left shoulder and the middle finger of the right hand, following a viral infection. Cold aggravated his condition and rest and heat eased it.

The chiropractor examined in particular a trigger point in the muscle over the left shoulder blade which reproduced the neck, shoulder and finger pain. Treatment of the muscle problem and spinal adjustment as necessary soon relieved the pain.

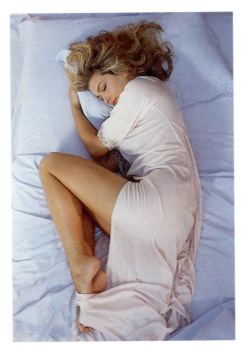 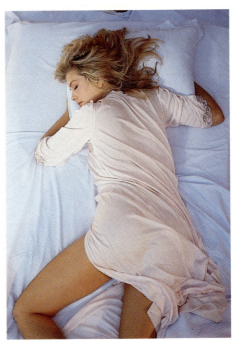

For a good night's rest it is essential firstly to sleep on a firm bed, and secondly to sleep in a good position. Lie on your back or side if possible; avoid lying on your stomach as this strains the neck and low back. Sufferers of severe back pain frequently find they are most comfortable curled up in the fetal position.

Postural habits at work can predispose someone to spinal stress. For example hairdressers or shop assistants who stand all day frequently get low back trouble. A hairdresser may also get problems with the neck and shoulders from repeatedly using the arms at awkward angles. People working at typewriters or desktop computers, where the desk is not high enough, or when the seat does not give enough support to the back, all provide examples of sources of mechanical stress and trauma that can lead to biomechanical problems in the spine. Badly designed furniture, either for children at school or adults both at work and at home – desks, chairs, beds, sofas and armchairs – can also cause spinal strain which in turn leads to back problems.

Bad posture and being overweight can cause postural distortions that lead to areas of spinal stress and eventual joint fixation problems. They can also arise from the presence of scoliosis – involving a weakening of the spine at certain levels. The presence of spinal asymmetries (in which, for example, the vertebrae may be fused on one side but not on the other), or having one leg shorter than the other, can also lead to localized stress on the spine.

The normal double-curvature of the spine is not the best shape for a creature that walks upright, and as a result human beings have a natural predisposition to mechanical strain in the back. There are slight weaknesses where the spine is most curved, which are susceptible to injury and can be aggravated by bad posture or clumsy lifting. Another type of mechanical trauma results when additional strain is put on the spine from a weakness in one of the joints in the legs – hip, knee or ankle – which makes a person walk with the body weight distributed unevenly.

Chemical irritants   Muscles that are not used regularly soon deteriorate, and the maintenance of muscle tone is essential for overall good health.

Biomechanical changes in the tissues can cause chronic and acute excessive tone (hypertonicity) or insufficient tone (hypotonicity) of the muscular system. These changes may in turn cause symptoms such as ischaemia (resulting from poor blood supply), anoxia (resulting from poor oxygen supply) and toxicity (the accumulation of poisonous wastes) in the tissues. The possible causes include nutritional deficiencies, smoking, exposure to harmful chemicals (by breathing or swallowing them), infection by micro-organisms (causing toxicity), exposure to excessive heat or cold, electric shock, foreign bodies in the tissues, ingestion of irritants (such as food that is too acidic or too alkaline), bad food combinations and food allergies.

Because the musculoskeletal system and the internal organs are closely interlinked through the nervous system, irritants that effect the internal organs can thus also affect the musculoskeletal system.

Psychological trauma   Most people do not fully realize what effects psychological stress and trauma can have on the physical body. We all know about stress causing problems such as ulcers, heart attacks, angina and even headaches and migraine. Less well known is that any type of psychological stress or shock can also affect the body physically to produce musculoskeletal tension and joint fixation, eventually giving rise to back pain, neck pain or chronic tension in the upper back and across the shoulders. Such psychological trauma can come from a variety of causes, such as overwork or worry. For chiropractic treatment to be effective in such cases, the cause of the stress also needs to be remedied.

Chiropractic adjustment in practice

We have described the biomechanical approach of a chiropractor to muscle and joint disorders and the aims of chiropractic therapy. But how is it done?

Many people think that when chiropractors treat the spine they are 'putting vertebrae back in place'. Strictly, vertebrae do not actually 'move out of place' in a literal sense; nevertheless their dynamics and functions are disturbed and the aim of the adjustment is to restore the spine's normal dynamics and anatomical and physiological functioning. To summarize the points covered so far, with regard to the different types of static and kinetic joint fixations, the aim of the chiropractor is:

● *To restore the spine to its normal position.*
● *To restore normal movement to an excessively mobile or extremely restricted part of the spine.*
● *To restore and correct a combination of these.*

The overall objective is to restore normal mechanical functioning to an area, so that other undesirable effects – brought about through the nervous and vascular systems – can be reduced.

The detailed effects of spinal manipulation of adjustment are not yet completely understood and, because most of them occur at a microscopic level in the spine, they are somewhat complicated to explain.

What is known for sure is that within the spinal cord there is a certain area that controls the transmission of sensory information, such as that concerning pain, touch, temperature and so on. The transmission of pain can be affected by changing the amount of other sensory input. For example, if you injure yourself you automatically rub the area. The proprioceptive nerve endings in the tissue are stimulated and send more impulses into the spinal cord. When this happens you feel less pain. It follows that any therapy bringing about more movement to the joints will at the same time help to inhibit the transmission of pain. It has also been shown that stretching the joint capsules inhibits those nerve pathways that are responsible for an increase in muscle excitability and muscle spasm.

The aim of manipulation is therefore to break the cycle of pain, muscle spasm and loss of movement that occurs in many spinal problems. Once this cycle is broken, healing and a return to normal function can begin. The intention is not only to return the joint function to normal but also to correct any abnormalities in the muscles, nerves, veins or lymph system.

Diagnostic and analytic techniques

We have discussed the importance of specific adjustments to restore normal biomechanics to the spine. But how does a chiropractor assess the spine in order to determine, specifically, which vertebra or vertebrae require adjustment?

The art of the chiropractor lies in this area of treatment especially. It relies on various analytical techniques combined with the refined sensitivity that chiropractors develop in their fingertips. They use this sensitivity to locate precisely the specific areas of the spine that they think are causing the patient's problem.

A chiropractor begins her analysis by taking the patient's

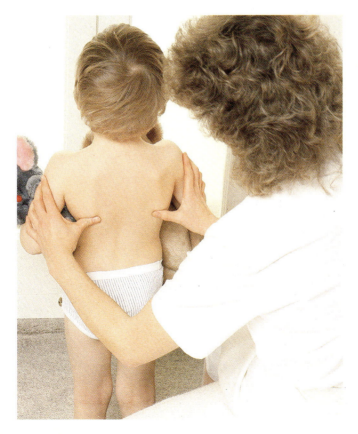

Spinal check ups can begin at any age – the earlier the better, so that any spinal problems can be detected and corrected before they develop into chronic problems later in life.

case history – a full and detailed account of the patient's state of health up to the time of the consultation, including any previous forms of treatment. The history is extremely important and can take the chiropractor much of the way along the road to a preliminary diagnosis. This can then be modified and clarified by various examination techniques until a final diagnosis is made. While the case history is being taken, the chiropractor has probably already observed how the patient walks, stands and sits, and has taken note of any unusual postural habits.

The chiropractor then examines the patient in the standing, sitting and lying positions. While the patient is standing, his or her general posture is noted – is the back long in comparison to the overall height, is the pelvis level or is one side higher than the other, are the shoulders level, is the head held upright or tilted to one side? Any changes to the normal spinal curves are

The chiropractor checks the general posture of the patient in order to detect any weakness or asymmetry (difference from one side to the other).

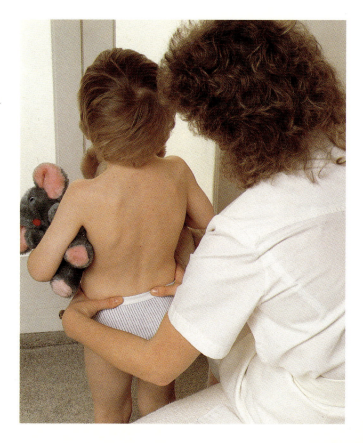

also noted – a straightening or an increase in the normal curve to the neck, rounded shoulders, and so on. A marked increase to the normal curve in the low back can shift the patient's centre of gravity and put extra stress on the bottom of the spine in the lumbo-sacral area, as well as on the vertebral facet joints. The chiropractor also checks for any signs of sideways curvature (scoliosis).

While the patient is still standing, he or she is asked to bend from side to side, flex forwards, arch backwards and turn from side to side by rotating at the hips. The chiropractor observes the patient's spine as it goes through these movements, so getting an idea of the location of any potential problems. The patient may then be asked to walk up and down so that the chiropractor can check the walking gait.

Next the patient is asked to sit on a chair so that the chiropractor can use a technique called motion palpation.

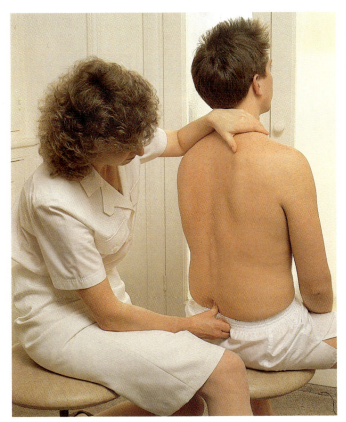

Motion palpation is an important diagnostic tool to the chiropractor. It is used to detect any alteration to the normal spine movement, whether it comes from a loss or an increase in the mobility of the joints.

Motion palpation

This technique is used to examine areas of the spine where there is a restricted amount of vertebral movement and joint play, or where there is excessive movement in the joint (hypermobility).

The patient's spine is taken through a series of movements while the chiropractor uses her fingers to palpate or feel the spinal joints to detect any abnormal areas. Each joint is felt individually while the spine is taken through the various movements of flexion and extension, rotation, and bending from side to side. In total there are some 115 joints in the spine that can be affected by alteration to the normal spinal biomechanics. As the joints are taken through the various movements, the chiropractor can also feel how much 'give' or 'play' there is in them by springing and testing ('challenging') the joints while feeling them with her fingertips.

As a follow-up to motion palpation, the chiropractor may employ what is called static palpation in order to confirm and further localize the diagnosis.

Static palpation

This technique can be carried out with the patient sitting, lying (face up or face down) or standing, depending on which area of the spine is being examined. It involves the chiropractor feeling the spinal tissues with her fingertips, and challenging and springing the vertebrae to determine the amount of give in the joints.

When there is an area of joint hypermobility or hypomobility, the overlying muscle and other soft tissue is usually also affected and its texture can change quite markedly. For instance, the chiropractor may be able to feel swelling in the tissue, perhaps accompanying inflammation. Sometimes the texture of the muscle changes, depending on how long it has been in spasm or under strain; with prolonged strain the muscle can become quite 'stringy' in nature. The patient may think that he or she has had a back problem for only one or two months, but when the chiropractor palpates the area he can tell whether or not there has been an underlying problem there, perhaps for many months or even years.

Depending on the texture of the muscle, the chiropractor can also detect areas of tenderness which usually accompany joint problems. In some cases, the tenderness is very painful, especially when the condition is acute. Static palpation also allows the chiropractor to find her way around the patient's

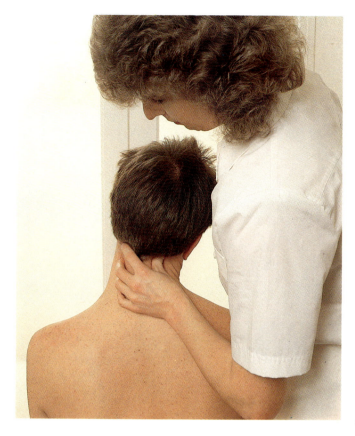

The chiropractor has a highly developed sense of touch in the fingertips which enables her to detect minute changes to joint mobility or in the texture of the soft tissue, which all help to indicate the source of the patient's pain problem.

spine. She can then note any changes of the normal outlines of the vertebrae, which may indicate an area of underlying stress.

Motion and static palpation can also be carried out on any other joints in the body, for example the knee or elbow, foot or ankle, hand or wrist. Palpation is therefore a very flexible and useful diagnostic tool for a chiropractor.

Orthopaedic and neurological examination

As part of her examination of the patient, the chiropractor also employs general orthopaedic and neurological tests of the kind used by orthodox medical practitioners. These tests help the chiropractor to confirm or eliminate certain types of conditions that could be implicated by the diagnosis, the patient's history and the pain he or she feels. In some cases these tests also help to monitor the patient's improvement as treatment progresses.

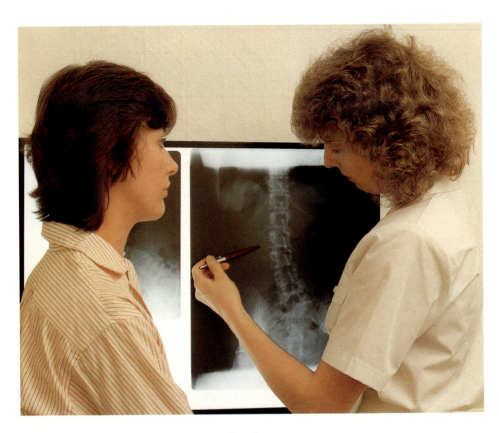

Most patients find that an explanation of their X-rays helps them to understand their back problems better. Chiropractors will generally discuss their X-ray findings with the patient prior to beginning treatment.

X-ray examination

If it is necessary – and safe for the patient – the chiropractor may X-ray an area of the spine. There may be a number of reasons that make this necessary. For instance, the chiropractor may suspect that there is an underlying pathological problem such as a fracture or infection, which needs to be confirmed or eliminated from the diagnosis. Many spines 'feel' quite normal from the outside, but X-rays reveal areas of considerable degenerative change. These can be in the intervertebral discs, in the spinal joints, or in both. They are sometimes accompanied by changes in the shape of the vertebrae, as a self-defence mechanism to protect that part of the spine. The changes can be much more severe than indicated by the case history or the examination, and can modify the treatment programme and ultimate prognosis of the condition.

The chiropractor also examines the X-rays for evidence of

areas of fixations and alterations to the normal shape and positioning of the vertebrae. This helps to determine which areas of the spine may need adjusting.

Once all the examination procedures have been completed, the chiropractor can fit together all the pieces of the jigsaw and make a diagnosis of the cause of the patient's disorder. And once she has identified the area of the spine or joints that are the likely cause of the problem, with due care and attention the chiropractor can begin treatment.

Chiropractic therapy

As earlier sections have explained, the main type of chiropractic treatment involves spinal or joint adjustment. This is frequently accompanied by soft-tissue massage to the area concerned. Because many spinal complaints are biomechanical in nature, it is obvious that some form of mechanical means should be applied to correct the mechanical problem. Chiropractic adjustment is just such a therapy. The examination methods aim to find out the cause of the problem before treatment begins, and then the treatment is directed at that particular cause.

Chiropractors do not prescribe drugs or carry out surgical procedures. Indeed, it is precisely because they use a natural form of treatment that many people seek their services, rather than those of their family doctor or hospital consultant. Many patients tell their chiropractors that they do not want to take drugs simply to relieve their symptoms. Pain exists, after all, to tell a person that something is wrong. Taking painkilling drugs deadens the pain temporarily, but the cause of the problem remains.

Drugs, by the very nature of the way they work, do not zero in on a specific cause or help to locate or diagnose it. Most drugs have effects on a much greater area of the body than the specific area of pain or disease for which they have been prescribed. And in addition there are always possible difficulties with the side-effects of drugs, which may add further problems to the ones the patient already has.

Although there are cases of surgical operations on the spine that have gone wrong, there are far more such operations that are totally successful. In some cases an operation is imperative and should not be delayed for any reason. An example is a severe disc collapse or protrusion which produces severe neurological complications. Nevertheless, because of the uncertain nature of spinal injuries, the outcome of many spinal

Everyone needs to find an exercise which best suits them and which they enjoy in order to help combat the onset of back and joint problems or mental stress and tension. Joggers should always make sure to wear the correct footwear to minimize the strain on the spine.

operations is doubtful and cannot be guaranteed. In these circumstances, many people consult a chiropractor first, before finally allowing a surgeon to operate, so that surgery is kept as a last resort.

Chiropractors see many patients who have, in fact, already received spinal surgery – some of which has succeeded, some of which has failed. Happily, a chiropractor can often help such cases. The types of manipulative techniques used are modified when treating the area around a surgical operation.

A common surgical procedure for persistent back trouble is an operation to fuse two or more vertebrae together. One of the problems with such spinal fusion, however, is that the patient tends to develop areas of increased mobility and wear and tear years later, usually above or below the area of the operation. These go on to cause spinal discomfort and pain of their own, for which the patient frequently consults a chiropractor.

The role of exercise

We are continually being told that exercise is good for us, and – within reason – this is true. Excess of any sort can be dangerous, and this applies as much to exercise as to other activities. However, everyone should exercise in some way. Furthermore, everyone can exercise in some way, be they disabled, confined to a wheelchair or just suffering with a bad back.

Exercise is important in the overall treatment regime of the chiropractor, but depends a great deal on the co-operation of the patient concerned. Many patients exercise regularly at first to speed up the healing process. But once their back feels better, they stop taking regular exercise and then of course the back problem returns.

Many of today's lifestyles include little, if any, exercise – although this seems to be changing rapidly. An increasingly large proportion of occupations involve sitting or standing inactively most of the day. Both tire the spine and strain it unduly. Even people in manual jobs are probably not exercising the spine healthily but instead are straining it unhealthily. A chiropractor will almost always advise a patient to undertake an exercise regime suited to his or her needs.

The start of a back problem is not necessarily the ideal time to start an exercise programme, however. The patient should keep mobile, but the back problem may be too acute to benefit from exercise. For this reason, the introduction of exercise into

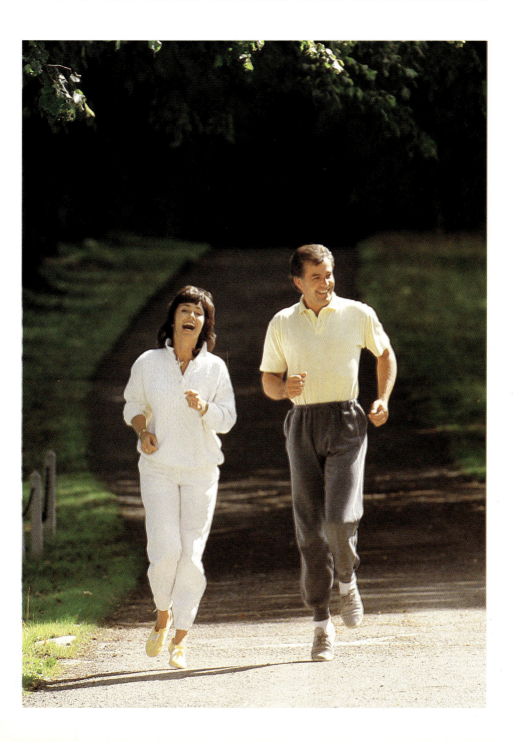

Severe back pain sufferers frequently find this an excellent way of relieving their pain either during the day at home or at night after work. This position allows the spine to relax and relieves the pressure on the disc joints.

the overall treatment regime has to be timed very carefully. Although back problems can often be traced to general lack of exercise and a resultant lack of overall muscle tone, unfortunately there is not one type of exercise that will benefit everyone equally, and so each person needs to be advised on an individual basis. Thus the type of exercises that are recommended can be tailored to the type of back problem the patient is suffering from.

Initially the patient may need various gentle stretching exercises in order to loosen up the spine. If these can be tolerated, then the patient can advance perhaps to exercises related to specific muscle groups. Commonly people who are

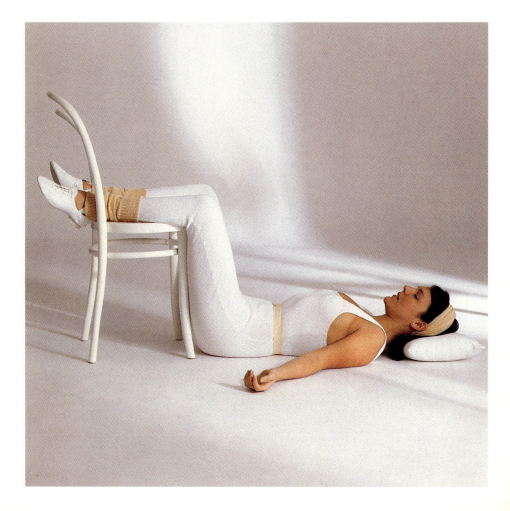

not keen on exercise stop there. Other patients may like to progress to more strenuous exercise, such as regular walking, swimming or cycling, which can usually be tolerated by most people without any ill effects.

The chiropractor therefore advises the patient about the type of exercise which would suit his or her particular back condition. Co-operation from the patient is, of course, essential for progress, although regrettably many patients do not seem eager to help themselves.

Whatever your views about exercise, however, the one thing to remember above all else is that, when exercises are done, there should be a sufficient warm-up period and the exercises should be carried out on a regular basis – for instance daily or three to four times a week.

Preventive measures

The chiropractor realizes better than anyone the need for good advice about preventing the re-occurrence of a spinal problem. Prevention should start both at home and at work. If the chiropractor asks questions about the patient's lifestyle, she is not merely being nosey, but is trying to visualize a complete picture of the patient's spine as it is put through its paces on a day-to-day basis. Because every different type of job has its own areas of stress and strain, by understanding and relating to that job as applied to the patient's spine, the chiropractor can offer individual advice on preventive measures to help that particular spine in that particular job.

The most obvious preventive measures are those involving chairs, seats and beds. Most people are probably aware of the importance of firm beds, chairs and upright seats in helping to prevent spinal problems. This is as true of a car seat as it is of a chair at work or in the home, and all should be taken into consideration.

Chiropractors also understand that it is not always easy for a person to adapt his work environment to suit his spine. Nevertheless they can only give what seems to be the best advice at the time – and this may often involve the patient changing aspects of his or her way of life. Nervousness about changing patterns of behaviour and anxiety about what others may say are common to all of us. On the other hand, a bad back is quite definitely the patient's problem alone, so a sensible patient will listen to what the chiropractor has to say about preventive measures and will act accordingly, regardless of what he or she imagines others may think.

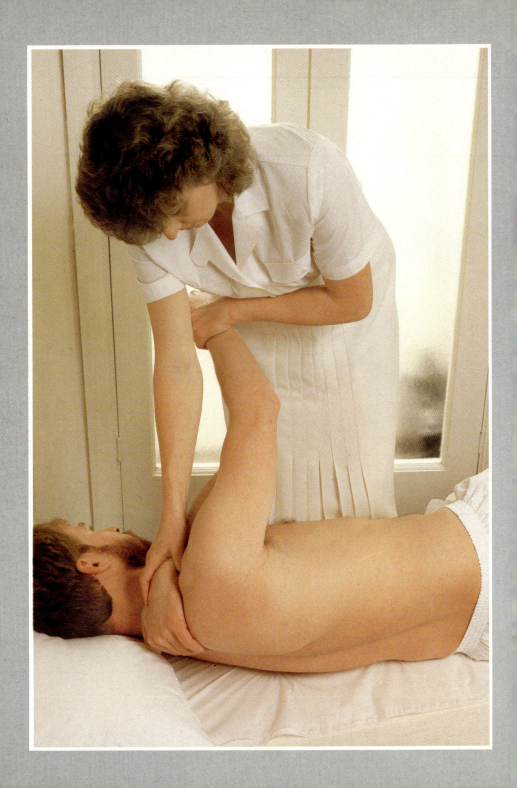

5

CHIROPRACTIC
IN ACTION

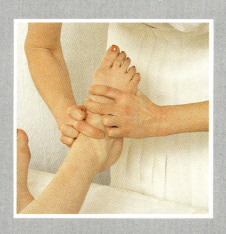

Before consulting a chiropractor it is usually necessary to make an appointment, and this is simply done by telephoning the clinic. When you visit the clinic for the first time, the receptionist will probably make a note of your name, address, telephone number and so on, and may also ask you your date of birth and occupation. In some clinics, you may be given a health questionnaire to fill out. You will then be shown to a seat in the waiting room until the chiropractor is ready to see you. Once the chiropractor is free, you will be shown through to the consultation room and introduced.

The chiropractor begins the consultation by asking various questions that enable her to compile a case history. She will inquire about the problem that has made you want to see her, which nearly always involves some sort of pain. But the extent and type of pain can vary a great deal. The chiropractor will want to know exactly where it hurts, how far the pain travels and the kind of pain it is. For example, is it restricted to one area, such as the low back or the neck, or does it spread down the legs or into the arms? Is the pain severe and sharp or dull and nagging like a toothache? In some cases the pain may be associated with or replaced by numbness or a pins and needles in the legs or arms.

The chiropractor will want to know how long you have been suffering with this particular problem – did it start last week, last month or last year? It is possible that it has existed for many years, and if so the chiropractor should be told. Or the problem may have just arisen, or it may be a recurrence of one that has been coming and going for some time; it is important that the chiropractor knows this as well.

She will also want to know if the pain is continuous or intermittent. For instance, it may be absent in the morning but come on and get worse as the day goes on, or be worse at night and in the morning, but ease off during the day. Also what aggravates or relieves the pain? For example, is it better or worse when you are sitting, standing or lying? Does coughing aggravate the pain, or does bending and leaning worsen it or ease it? Have you tried applying heat or ice to the area and does it help or make things worse? Have you noticed that anything else aggravates it, such as sitting at a desk all day? Your answers to these questions are important to the chiropractor because they enable her to construct a complete picture not only of your problem but also of the characteristics of your lifestyle that may have a bearing on her diagnosis.

There are other questions as well. What was the initial cause

Out of the blue It is not unusual for a new patient, usually male, to be sitting opposite the chiropractor explaining the history of his back problem and declaring that it all started 'out of the blue'. One look at him slouching in his chair in what is obviously his natural sitting posture tells the chiropractor exactly what has caused the problem. A little more care would have saved him the chiropractor's consultation fee!

WHAT THE CHIROPRACTOR ASKS

When you consult a chiropractor, be prepared to answer the following typical diagnostic questions:

- Where does it hurt?
- Does the pain spread to other parts of the body?
- How long have you had the pain?
- Is it continuous or intermittent?
- What sort of pain is it? Sharp, aching, dull, numb, pins and needles?
- Do you know why the problem began?
- Have you ever had this pain before? If so when? How did it start? How long did it last?
- Does anything aggravate the pain? Or ease it? If so, what?
- Does the pain stop you sleeping at night?
- Are you stiff in the morning?
- Is the pain better or worse when you sit? Stand? Walk?
- Have you had any previous treatment?
- If so, was it effective?
- How is your general health?
- Have you any history of falls? Accidents? Serious illness?
- Operations?
- Do you take regular exercise?
- Is there anything you would like to add?

of the problem? Did it occur suddenly or did it come on after lifting something, bending down, sitting all day, or driving a long way in a car? In some cases the onset of a problem cannot be tied in to any specific occurrence – but if this is the case it may be significant so the chiropractor wants to know that as well.

Previous treatment The chiropractor will want to know if you have already been treated for the condition. If so, what type of treatment have you received? Whom did you consult? Did the treatment help? What was the diagnosis made by your doctor or specialist, and did he send you for any X-rays, blood tests or any other sort of tests? If so, do you know the results?

General health Your general state of health is also relevant to the chiropractor. Are you being treated for any other health problem? If so, what is it and what type of treatment are you receiving? Have you a history of any serious illnesses or operations? If so, what were they?

Past history Many patients totally forget about their past histories of serious illness, operations or accidents at the initial visit. Then at the second session they casually remark that they've had some organ or other removed or that five years ago they fell down a flight of stone steps. All chiropractors are used to this exasperating selective memory!

Falls and other accidents The chiropractor will want to know if you have had any falls or accidents – for instance a car accident. If so, what were they and when did they occur?

Family health Do any health problems run in your family? If so, what are they? This can also be extremely important.

Drugs Are you taking any type of medication at the present time? If so, do you know their names and what you are taking them for? Also, how long have you been on the drugs?

Some of these questions may seem irrelevant at first, but they all help the chiropractor to build up a picture of you and your problem, and the case history contributes a great deal to making a diagnosis of your condition. In some instances it takes 30 minutes or more for the chiropractor to obtain all the details she needs. In others, which are more straightforward, it may take only ten minutes or so. Very often, the initial cause of a back or neck problem may not be known. Then the chiropractor may well ask for quite a few details about your lifestyle and the type of work you do, as well as asking about any sports you play or any hobbies in which you participate. The chiropractor is not merely being nosy – all of these queries help her towards her final diagnosis.

The examination
Once the case history has been taken, the chiropractor usually asks you to undress to your underwear. Back–fastening gowns, allowing easy access to the spine, are usually provided.

Examination of the neck This is carried out for problems involving the neck, shoulders or arms, and for headaches and migraine. The chiropractor will ask you to sit on a stool or in a chair. She usually first applies a number of orthopaedic and neurological tests – similar to those that a doctor or specialist would make – to check the function of the nerves and bones. If all is not in order, a positive test helps with the final diagnosis.

Once these tests have been done, the chiropractor checks the general movements of the neck by asking you to bend your head forwards, backwards and from side to side, and to turn your head from side to side. The chiropractor can see if there is any limitation to the normal movement of the neck, and she is also able to tell if any of these movements are painful. Next the chiropractor uses her fingertips to feel the bones and muscles in

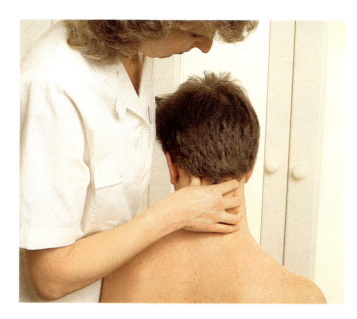

When examining the neck, the chiropractor will use her fingers to gently palpate or feel the movement of the vertebrae in the neck and to check the amount of muscle tension and ligament strain in the area. This will all help her to arrive at a final diagnosis.

in the neck, to check for any areas of increased muscle spasm or even inflammation. She can also feel the alignment of the bones and whether this is normal or otherwise.

Then, still with her fingers feeling the neck, the chiropractor moves the neck forwards and backwards, bends it from side to side, and turns the head to look for any parts of the spine in which the vertebrae are not moving freely or perhaps are even moving too freely. This enables the chiropractor to locate the area of the spine that could be the cause of the problem.

If necessary, the chiropractor repeats this procedure in the upper part of the back, because neck disorders are often accompanied by problems in the upper back and shoulder area as well.

The chiropractor may, at times, ask if this or that point is tender, and in any case you as the patient should tell her if any areas she touches feels sore or painful. Usually, however, the chiropractor can detect whether a particular place is sore by the feel of it, without you having to tell her.

While you are in a sitting position, the chiropractor can also examine your shoulders, taking each joint in turn through its various movements, to see whether there is any restriction at the joint and if there is pain in the shoulder. The chiropractor can also palpate, or feel, all round the soft tissues in the shoulders to check for any damage or tender spots in the muscles.

Instant cures Some people hear such good things about chiropractors that they expect them to have 'magic hands' and to be completely cured in one treatment session. Such people frequently become quite annoyed when the chiropractor insists on taking a detailed case history, examination and possibly X-rays before making a diagnosis and starting treatment. Very occasionally an almost miraculous recovery can happen, but this is very rare and only occurs in very specific types of spinal problems.

The chiropractor looks at the spine as a whole to assess the posture of the patient and checks the levels of the height of the shoulder blades and the pelvis to determine any inequalities from one side to the other. Few of us are completely symmetrical and inequalities can contribute to back problems.

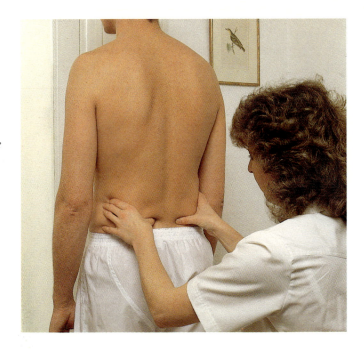

Examination of the low back This can sometimes be a more lengthy procedure than examination of the neck. First, the chiropractor usually asks you to stand with your back towards her so that she can look at your spine. She then checks the shape of your back – are the spinal curves normal or are they altered in any way? Is the pelvis level or is it tilted because one leg is shorter than the other? Are the shoulders level? While you are standing, the chiropractor may ask you to bend forwards, arch your spine backwards slightly, and bend from side to side. Again she will check for any areas of restricted movement and see if any of the movements are painful or not.

The chiropractor will probably then ask you to sit on a stool or on the edge of the treatment table and, feeling with her fingertips, take the spine through its various range of motions to check for any areas where the spinal movement is restricted or hypermobile.

Then the chiropractor will need you to lie down on the treatment table, first face up and then face down, and carry out various orthopaedic and neurological tests, which will again help her to eliminate or confirm a possible diagnosis. When this is done the chiropractor may make you lie face down on the treatment table so that she can palpate your back while you

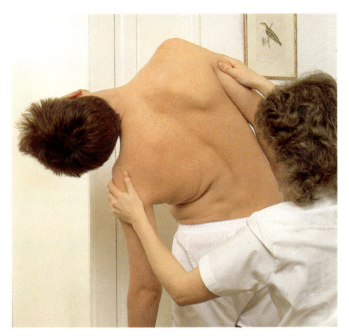

The chiropractor will ask the patient to bend his spine in various directions: from side to side, forward and backwards as far as is comfortably possible, in order to check the overall movement of the spine. When these movements are performed, the chiropractor can see any area which is not moving normally and which could be the source of the back problem.

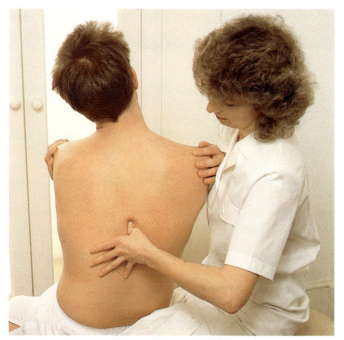

After the overall movement of the spine, the chiropractor checks the individual movements of the vertebrae by contacting the side of each vertebra, usually with a thumb, and moving the patient into various positions such as bending backwards and forwards (flexion), side bending (lateral bending), stretching (extension) and twisting (rotation). Those vertebrae that move too freely, or not freely enough can then be detected.

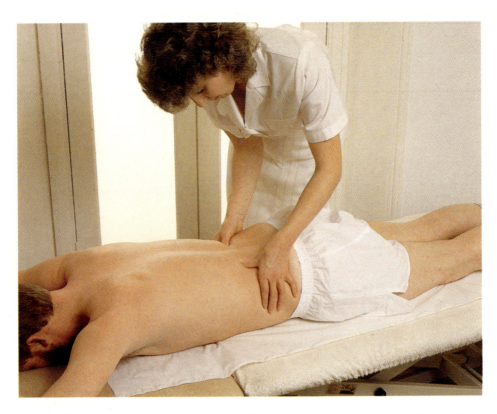

Once the chiropractor has checked the spinal and vertebral movement, she will also make a general check on the texture and tension of the soft tissue, that is the muscle tendons and ligaments overlying the spine.

are in a neutral and non–weight-bearing position. She can then feel any area in the spine where there is tenderness, an increase in muscle spasm or a change in texture of the muscle. All this helps her to locate the part of the spine that could be causing the problem and the associated pain. While you are in this position, the chiropractor can in fact check the whole of the spine.

It should be mentioned that the exact procedure may vary from chiropractor to chiropractor because each has his or her own way of examining a patient; what has been described here is, however, typical. The examination can also vary depending on the condition of the patient.

Some patients are in so much pain that many of the examination procedures cannot be carried out immediately, and the chiropractor has to administer a type of 'first aid' treatment in order to reduce the severity of the condition. But in these types of problems, the diagnosis is usually much more obvious than in longer standing, chronic conditions.

Examination of the hands and feet   If you are consulting a chiropractor because of a problem with a knee, ankle or wrist, it may be necessary to undress only sufficiently to expose the part concerned. But sometimes such disorders are associated with underlying spinal problems – for instance, neck trouble affecting the elbows and wrist or low back trouble for the knee and ankle. Therefore do not be surprised if the chiropractor asks you to undress so that she can examine your spine as well.

During all these examination procedures, the chiropractor is continually thinking about what she has learned from you in the case history and what she has picked up during the examination, so that she can diagnose the cause of your problem. Sometimes it is not so straightforward and there could be more than one possible cause – and for this reason the chiropractor may continue to ask further and perhaps quite in-depth questions. There is always a reason for this. Even questions concerning bowel movements and bladder function can have particular relevance in cases of low back pain.

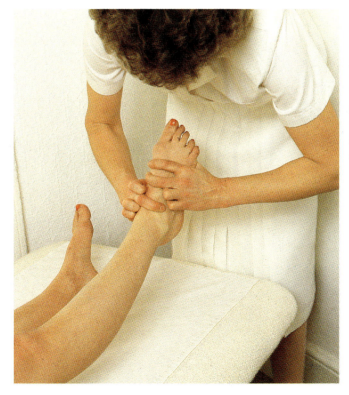

The chiropractor is not limited to the examination or treatment of the spinal problems, but can also examine, diagnose and treat extremity joint problems as well. Here the chiropractor is preparing to adjust a foot problem.

X-raying the patient

X-ray photographs, particularly of the spine, are an extremely useful diagnostic tool that chiropractors use for the overall benefit of the patient. But not every patient needs to be X-rayed. Whether or not this is done depends on a number of factors. For example, pregnant women are not X-rayed at all, and women of child-bearing age are only X-rayed during the ten days following the start of a menstrual period (to prevent any possibility of radiation damage to a fetus). In some cases, although the examination does not lead to a clear diagnosis,

X-rays are an important part of the diagnostic procedure used by the chiropractor. Not every patient will need them, but in many cases X-rays will help the chiropractor in the final diagnosis and in ruling out any underlying problem where chiropractic manipulation may be contra-indicated. X-rays also give the chiropractor important structural information which can help to determine which type of techniques to use.

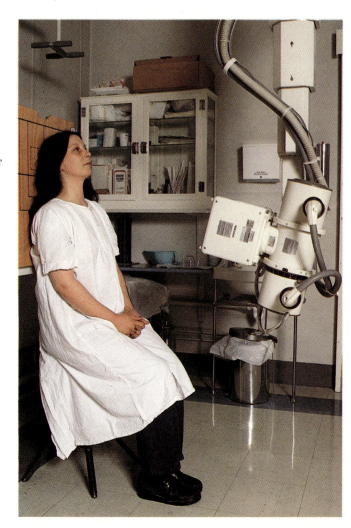

the X-rays may reveal the source of a problem. They may also help to detect disorders for which chiropractic is not necessarily the right sort of treatment, and the patient should be referred elsewhere.

X-ray examination also assists the chiropractor when she tries to make a prognosis for the condition. For example, the presence of severe degenerative changes in the spine of a farmer would indicate that his back problem is very likely to recur unless he takes more care while working. The state of the spine, the amount of degeneration or wear and tear, the shape of the curves and the density of the bones can all affect the type of manipulative treatment given by a chiropractor, and may indicate that she should modify the proposed treatment.

Making a diagnosis

The chiropractor has now reached the stage when she feels able to make her diagnosis. In some cases this may be very straightforward, whereas in others it is not so clear and a differential diagnosis may be necessary. For example, someone may be suffering with a low back problem, but the position of the pain is such that it could be a low back pain referred from a kidney disorder. Or in a woman there may be a history of trouble with her menstrual periods and the low back pain may be accompanied by abdominal pain. In this case, is the abdominal pain referred from the back or is it a symptom of a gynaecological problem which is itself causing the low back pain?

In more serious disorders, there may be signs that the back condition is caused by a bone infection or even some sort of tumour, in the bone or pressing on the spinal cord or a nerve.

In some cases the examination may not reveal any disorder at all in the spine and yet the pain is very real. Then the chiropractor has to try to decide where the pain is coming from, because the patient will need to return to his or her family doctor for further tests and examination. The gall bladder, for example, is well known for referring pain not only to the upper back, but also between the shoulder blades, in the shoulder and in the low back. The liver can refer pain to the right shoulder, and the heart can refer pain to the left arm. Stomach problems such as ulcers can also give severe pain in the upper back between the shoulder blades. All this needs to be taken into account before a final diagnosis can be made.

For these reasons, chiropractic treatment is not appropriate

Diagnostic points This is the order in which the chiropractor proceeds with a new patient:
● Where is the main source of the pain?
● Is there any referred pain? If yes, where does the pain go?
● What is the type of pain?
● Is it sharp, or dull achy?
● Is there numbness or pins and needles?
● What aggravates the condition?
● What eases the condition?
● Any past history of trouble?
● Any history of accidents
● Previous health history
● Previous treatment
● Examination findings
● X-ray findings
● Diagnosis; decision about whether to treat or not
● Treatment begins or patient is referred elsewhere.

for every patient a chiropractor sees. But the chiropractor seldom knows this until after she has completed the case history, made an examination and possibly taken X-rays.

On occasion it may be that the patient is asked to return to his or her family doctor or to visit a specialist for appropriate diagnosis and treatment, although at the same time some form of chiropractic treatment may also be viable. A good example is someone with arthritis in the hip joint. A chiropractor can diagnose this condition, and is able to tell whether or not the problem is severe enough to warrant an operation. If it is, the chiropractor will almost certainly refer the patient back to the family doctor for referral to an orthopaedic specialist. The orthopaedic specialist may then decide that an operation is necessary, but the waiting list for the operation may be lengthy. In such cases, the chiropractor can still treat the patient's hip problem in order to keep him or her mobile and relatively free from pain until surgery can be done.

There are other conditions that chiropractic treatment cannot cure but where such treatment can help to improve the quality of life of the sufferer. Examples include 'bamboo spine' (ankylosing spondylitis) a rheumatic infection which results in severe stiffness as the joints and ligaments between the vertebrae lose all flexibility and become almost bone-like, or a sufferer from multiple sclerosis or some other disabling disease who may be confined to a wheelchair and as a result suffer from low back or neck problems.

Chiropractic cannot cure cancer, but sometimes chiropractors are asked to help to improve the quality of the patient's life when spinal pain is involved. Obviously the chiropractor needs to understand fully the condition she is dealing with, so that she can make any appropriate adjustments to the treatment.

Chiropractic treatment

The consultation, examination and any X-rays usually occur on the first visit to the chiropractor. On the second visit, the chiropractor explains what she has learned from the examination and X-rays and says whether she feels that chiropractic treatment is viable for that particular case.

The chiropractor then outlines how she intends to proceed with the treatment and what the ultimate outcome of it is likely to be. Once this is done, treatment can start. Because there are about 36 different types of techniques, different chiropractors may approach the same problem in a number of ways. In general, however, treatment may progress as follows.

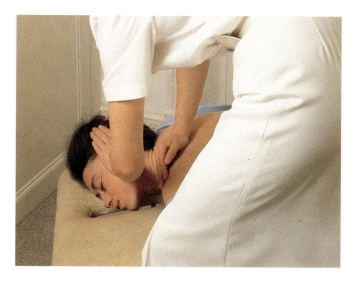

The chiropractor is able to use many different adjustive methods in order to manipulate the neck. This is just one of those techniques. In spite of the positioning, it is not a painful procedure in expert hands.

Treating the neck A chiropractor can treat the neck with the patient sitting or lying down (face up or face down). First she checks the spine to finally localize the area she feels requires adjustment, and often does some soft-tissue work on the area concerned to loosen up the muscles before adjusting the spine. The chiropractor then makes contact with the neck, using part of her hand, on the area she wishes to adjust. She stabilizes the other side of the neck or head with her hand and moves the head and neck so that they are in just such a position that a quick flick of the wrist will allow the chiropractor to adjust the spine. This movement is often accompanied by a cracking noise from the joint which can sound very loud to the patient. However the chiropractor usually warns the patient of what is about to happen so that he or she is not alarmed by these sudden cracking noises. The procedure may then be repeated elsewhere in the neck.

The chiropractor checks to see if she has achieved what she expected – that is, some alteration to the movement of the joints in the neck. Very often, the chiropractor does not attempt to do too much at the first treatment until she can assess how the patient reacts to it. Some patients react quite dramatically, others less so. And some can suffer severe reactions, especially if the chiropractor is trying to mobilize an area that has been restricted for a long time.

At this stage the chiropractor may advise the patient about certain dos and don'ts and preventive measures.

Treating the upper back This is done with the patient standing, sitting or, more commonly, lying face up or face down on the treatment table. Again, the chiropractor may first loosen up any muscle tension in the area and follow this with the chiropractic adjustment.

To adjust the spine, a chiropractor also takes a specific contact with one or both hands on the area of the spine concerned. The patient will then be asked to breathe in and out, and on the outward breath the chiropractor will thrust quickly down with the contact hand. This will adjust the spine in that area. Following treatment, the chiropractor continually reassesses the spine to see if she has achieved the required aim – to restore normal function to that part of the spine. She may repeat this manoeuvre on other vertebra until she is happy that the treatment has been effective.

The chiropractor is adjusting the middle of the upper back, using a different type of 'diversified' technique to that shown on page 60. Back pain in this area can sometimes lead to digestive problems.

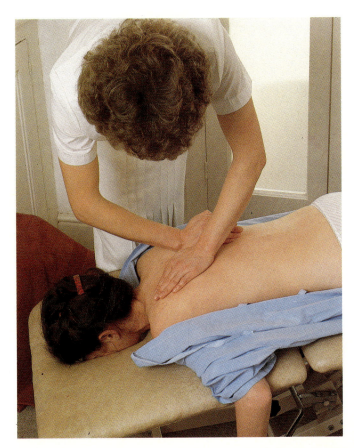

Treating the low back For this treatment, the patient may be asked either to sit or to lie down (face up, face down, or on one side). The most common positions for this type of low back adjustment are with the patient lying on one side, or face down on the treatment table.

Again the chiropractor may first prepare the low back before the adjustment by using some soft-tissue techniques on the muscles. Then she takes a specific contact with one hand on the part of the lumbar spine she wishes to adjust, and positions the patient's body in such a way that the vertebra can be adjusted with a quick thrust of the contact hand. The adjustment is again often accompanied by an audible click, and the procedure may be repeated elsewhere in the patient's lumbar spine. Following the adjustment the chiropractor reassesses the spinal movement.

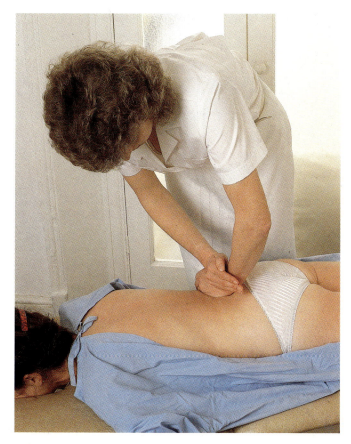

Here the chiropractor is adjusting the low back, using a 'toggle-recoil' technique. This is quite different to other techniques in that the patient will always be lying face down on the table.

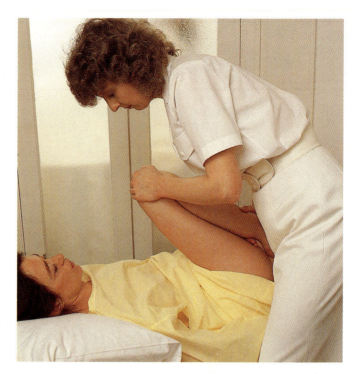

The chiropractor here is treating a hip problem using general mobilization techniques as part of the overall treatment.

It is quite common for more than one area of the spine to be treated during a single visit to the chiropractor, especially if the patient is suffering from both a low back problem and a neck problem. Every chiropractor has his or her own particular techniques for adjusting the spine, and so you could visit a number of them who would all be attempting to achieve the same thing, but doing it in different ways. Obviously the chiropractor's physical build as well as that of the patient will to some extent determine the types of techniques used, because some require more force than others.

The amount of time a treatment takes also varies. Some treatments last only 5 to 10 minutes, others 20 to 30 minutes, depending on the complexity of the situation. Some chiropractors prefer to work more slowly and chat more to their patients, because it is less tiring for them. Others can achieve exactly the same results by working faster and chatting less! Whichever way your chiropractor works, remember that this type of therapy is very tiring for the practitioner. All chiropractors have different ways of practising, depending on their own physique and physical fitness.

Subsequent treatment

At subsequent consultations the treatment is likely to be similar to the first visit. Initially the chiropractor asks the patient how he or she has fared since the last treatment – was there a reaction to it, did it aggravate the condition, did it ease it, or was there merely no change?

The chiropractor then re-examines the spine to see if, using palpation, she can detect any changes, and if so she may modify the treatment accordingly. With some treatments the chiropractor expects certain improvements, and whether or not these have occurred tells her how much the technique she is using is likely to help that patient. If there is no change, the chiropractor reassesses the situation and advises the patient accordingly.

Sometimes the chiropractor needs to use certain adjuncts to help the treatment – such as the application of heat, cold, ultra-sound or other medical techniques. The main source of treatment, however, will always come from the chiropractor's hands.

Treatments for acute and chronic conditions

Occasionally the patient is in such pain, or in such an acute condition for other reasons, that the chiropractor is unable to examine him fully or to take X-rays. If this is the case, she will carry out certain types of treatment immediately in order to settle the pain and ease the situation. She will obviously make sure that any treatment given at this stage is safe for the patient. Subsequently, when the pain has subsided sufficiently, the chiropractor can proceed with the rest of the examination and X-rays, perhaps at the next consultation.

A patient who has suffered with back trouble for some time is not usually given immediate treatment. In such cases the chiropractor often waits until after she receives the X-ray results before commencing therapy. Sometimes the chiropractor also needs time to consider all aspects of the patient's condition before she can make a diagnosis and plan a treatment regime, because not all back problems are easy to diagnose or straightforward to treat.

Once treatment has commenced, the chiropractor proceeds at a pace suited to each individual patient, which she may have to adapt and change as therapy progresses. Some patients expect immediate relief and miraculous recovery rates, even though they may have suffered with the back problem for many years. It does not help the patient if he or she tries to

Casenote Mr R suffered with an acute onset (five days) of low back pain with sciatica (pins and needles) in the right leg. When he consulted the chiropractor he was antalgic (leaning to one side) and the chiropractor was hardly able to examine the spine as all movements produced severe pain. Fortunately, Mr R was able to lie face down on the treatment table and receive pain relieving treatment so that the chiropractor could later begin more active therapy.

Mr R's condition started after he had lifted a heavy bag of coal, and was a recurrence of an old disc problem. Initial treatment would include an ice regime for him to do at home (ice packs on the back) in order to help reduce inflammation.

persuade the chiropractor to give him more treatment than is suitable at any one time. After all, the chiropractor is the expert and knows what should be done.

Different types of treatment

The 36 main types of chiropractic techniques have various names. Diversified, Gonstead, SOT, Applied Kinesiology and Toggle-Recoil are some practised in Britain and the USA.

To help with treatment most chiropractors use a specially designed chiropractic table – made up of a number of movable parts which make the job that much easier for the therapist and more comfortable for the patient. Many people are worried that chiropractic treatment will be painful. It is not the treatment that is painful, however, so much as the complaint from which the patient is suffering. All treatment is done within the pain limits of the patient, and if it hurts to adjust the spine in one direction, or using one method, the chiropractor can at least try another one which may well be less painful.

Chiropractors are thus very adaptable in their adjustive

Here the chiropractor is adjusting the child's neck. The techniques used to treat children are similar to those used to treat adults, but modified in such a way that the amount of force required to do the adjustment is reduced.

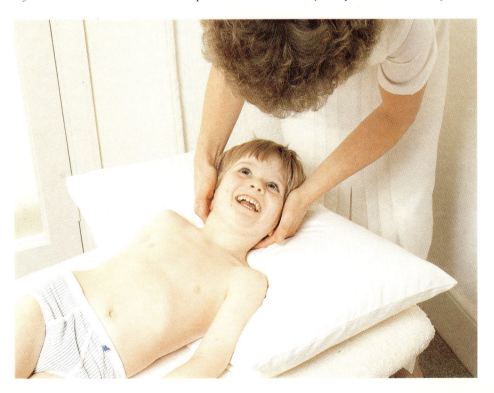

techniques. It must also be said that they need to be able to adapt, because the type of technique used to treat a baby is obviously different from that for a fit teenager, a stout rugby player or 70-year-old grandmother. It is because of this adaptability that chiropractic is able to treat such a wide range of problems in different age groups and in people of varying physiques.

Reactions to treatment

Each patient may react to manipulative treatment in a different way. Most reactions occur following the first one or two sessions. Some patients may feel no different at all until they have received several treatments. Others feel immediately better for a few hours or a day or so, and then regress back to the original pain. This may occur after a few treatments have been given, until their effects seem to last a bit longer each time.

In some patients the reaction may be to feel immediately worse for a day or so. When this type of reaction occurs, the problem usually settles down and the patient starts to recover. Some people even report that following manipulative treatment they can feel quite 'high' and full of energy, and they rush around doing far too much – but needless to say the next day they usually feel dreadful. On the other hand patients may report feeling very tired after treatment and in need of a good sleep. If the patient can lie down and go to sleep, he or she usually benefits from it and the results of the treatment are speedier.

All of these types of reactions can be regarded as normal. In 1972 the author Maigne classified reactions to manipulation in two ways: those that are painful and those that are functional. He described a number of different types of painful and functional reactions, which are also typical of those which a chiropractic patient may experience.

Painful reactions Following manipulation, 40 per cent of patients are said to suffer with diffuse pain which comes on fairly soon after treatment and lasts from six to eight hours. The reaction results from the release of strong adhesions around the joints and usually occurs after the first treatment; it is not so common after subsequent treatments.

Some patients complain of general muscular aches and pains following treatment, which may come on following a slight delay. They can then last from half a day to a week, but on average persist for only two or three days. This is apparently a

Casenote Miss Y had woken up six days previously with a stiff neck and had gradually developed a severe headache and lack of normal mental clarity. After examination, treatment of the neck began. Immediately after treatment Miss Y was able to move her neck, her headache disappeared and she felt extremely light-headed. She was instructed to go home and sleep for a couple of hours. Following this the problem completely cleared up.

good prognostic sign and occurs only following the first couple of treatments.

On occasion, after treatment a diffuse pain may start and last for more than two days, or there may be a temporary exaggeration of the original pain or a recurrence of it in an altered form. These different types of reactions can have specific meanings to the chiropractor and therefore the patient should report them when asked. It may be that the chiropractor will need to alter or modify the treatment in some way. Of course, if the reaction is very severe, or if the patient is at all worried, he or she should not hesitate to contact the chiropractor for advice.

Functional reactions   These are quite different from painful reactions and, when they occur, often seem unrelated to the spine. For instance, it is very common for the patient to start to perspire all over the trunk and under the armpits. This can start immediately the treatment is over and does not last long. This type of reaction arises from stimulation of the sympathetic nervous system, and is nothing to worry about.

If, in addition to a back problem, a patient complains of abdominal or pelvic pain, it can be aggravated following chiropractic treatment, although the pain does not necesarily start immediately. Again, there is rarely any need to worry, but never hesitate to consult your chiropractor if you are troubled by reactions of this sort.

Other possible reactions include episodes of general tremor with trembling and chills, diarrhoea, fainting, palpitation, cold and nausea. These reactions are uncommon, but they do happen, and if they occur let your chiropractor know.

Most reactions to treatment, therefore, occur following the first couple of sessions. The chiropractor usually modifies the treatment to reduce them. Sometimes, in order to start the repair process so that the back can return to normal function and the pain can subside, it is necessary for the patient to suffer an initial worsening of symptoms.

Advice on posture and exercises

As the treatment progresses, the chiropractor may start to advise the patient on how to help him or herself in the future, either to prevent a recurrence of a back or neck problem, or how to reduce any stresses in everyday life that might be contributing to it in the first place. Advice on posture and exercise may also be necessary at this stage.

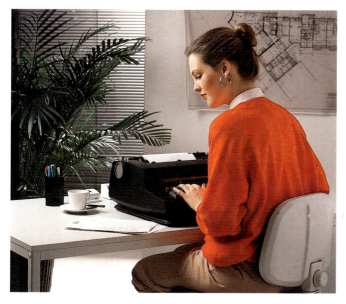

Secretaries frequently suffer from neck and shoulder problems as a result of sitting typing at desks all day. When the copy paper is placed to the side of the typewriter as here, the strain on the neck is increased, aggravating the problem. VDU and computer operators suffer with similar problems as well as from repetitive strain injuries to the wrists.

Posture This is important not only in the standing and walking positions but even more so when sitting down. Of all postures, the sitting one puts the most strain on the spine and is the single causative factor in a great many low back problems. A good sitting posture is therefore imperative, whether at work, driving a car or at home.

A good sitting posture requires a proper chair – that is, one which gives adequate support to the upper low back, low back, buttocks and thighs. If the chair fails to support any of these areas adequately, stresses can build up and back pain can result. You should check the chairs at home and choose one that best suits your needs. Often sofas and armchairs do not give adequate support for the back, and in some cases it is necessary to buy a special armchair that gives adequate comfort and proper support. If you sit all day at work, your chair is obviously of vital importance. Unfortunately most office chairs are bought for their cheapness or looks rather than for whether or not they are good for the back.

Few car seats ever suit their driver and most of us need to pad out the seat in some way. Those who regularly drive a considerable mileage are prone to low back and neck problems. It is essential that drivers stop regularly to exercise and stretch themselves. Not only does this help their backs, but the exercise can stimulate them in other ways, including mentally, and make them more alert on the road.

It should be evident to everyone how important a good standing posture is – with the shoulders back, the stomach pulled in and the buttocks tucked in as well. Not only does such a posture improve the back but it also stops the internal organs from getting squashed; the lungs can expand properly, you appear taller and psychologically it puts you in a better mood. It is interesting to note how much your posture can reflect your mood and how you feel about yourself; and from force of habit changing your posture seems to have a return effect on the way you feel.

Posture in bed can also be important. It is always better to lie on your back or on one side when sleeping. The fetal position – lying on one side with the knees drawn up – is particularly comfortable for back sufferers. People who habitually sleep on their stomachs frequently suffer with neck problems and headaches, and this sleeping position should definitely be discouraged.

A good sleeping position is important and back sufferers usually find lying on one side or the other more comfortable. Sometimes, specially designed neck pillows will also give comfort to those who spend the night wrestling with their pillows to find a bearable position for their necks.

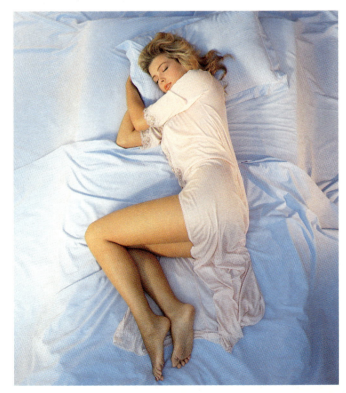

Prevention

Virtually every job can cause a spinal problem of some nature. There are no ideal jobs in life – ones that involve equal amounts of sitting, standing and walking around which can be interchanged on a regular basis throughout the working day. Most occupations involve too much sitting, too much standing, too much bending or too much walking around. Other jobs involve lifting, repetitive movements or working in awkward, twisted positions. Any and all of these can result in spinal problems of some type – be they low back or neck problems.

Your aim should be to try to modify the effects that job positions have on your back. By understanding the type of job a patient does, a chiropractor is able to suggest ways to help alter the various stresses and strains. For example, if the patient is a teacher bending over pupils' desks all day, can the pupils come to the teacher at his or her desk instead? If the patient is a farmer, does he habitually lift heavy loads alone when he should get help, or does he jump down from the tractor instead of climbing down? If the patient has a job that involves standing all day, is he or she wearing sensible shoes? They can have a heel, but are the soles such that they will help to absorb the strain? For example, shoes with soft crêpe soles are much better to stand in, and some people even find wearing a comfortable pair of trainers for work much better for their backs.

Because there are so many different types of jobs and work environments, advising each person on an individual basis needs considerable experience and expertise, combined with a chiropractor's understanding of the spine and the complicated way in which it works.

A good bed is another simple preventive measure. Most people are by now aware that you should have a bed that is comfortable yet firm enough to support the spine while you are asleep – one that does not sag but is not so hard that it feels like sleeping on a layer of concrete. If the bed is too soft it will strain the back; if it is too hard it may cause bruising. Nevertheless it is not necessary to spend a great deal of money to get a good bed. Most chiropractors can advise a patient on the best type of bed for his or her particular problems.

Young mothers frequently suffer with bad backs because of continual lifting and bending with babies and young children. All surfaces used to change nappies should be of a height that makes bending and leaning unnecessary. The baby should be

OCCUPATIONAL HAZARDS

Some jobs carry a risk of injury or problems in specific areas of the body.

Neck shoulder and arm problems **Wrist injuries**	Clerical workers Secretaries Computer/ VDU operators Journalists
Neck, shoulder and arm problems **Low back problems**	Hairdressers Sales representatives Car and lorry drivers Teachers
Low back problems	Manual workers Nurses Shop assistants Dentists Architects Engineers Gardeners Taxi drivers Pilots

lifted from the floor with your knees bent. It is not a good idea to sit the baby on one hip when standing, because this also strains the spine. Forethought and planning can help to avoid such problems.

Secretaries, typists and computer operators frequently suffer with neck problems, shoulder problems, headaches and even wrist disorders. These can result from sitting in a bad chair with a desk at the wrong height; looking to one side (the same side) all day while copy-typing; tensing yourself to hear what is being said when audio-typing; concentrating on a VDU without a break to rest the eyes; and repetitive strain injury to the wrists through frequent typing at the wrong angle or on a heavy manual keyboard. Modern electric and electronic typewriters considerably reduce the amount of stress and strain on the neck and shoulders while typing.

A chiropractor regards advice on prevention as a very important part of the overall treatment regime, and it makes a great difference when the patient actually heeds the advice!

Exercise

It cannot be overemphasized that exercise is essential for everyone whether he or she is fit or fat, able-bodied or disabled. There are very few people who cannot find some sort of exercise that suits them. For back sufferers, the safest type of exercises are generally acknowledged to be walking, swimming and cycling.

Walking   Many back sufferers are unable to walk far at first, but even starting with only five minutes a day and gradually building up to twenty minutes a day is beneficial. The aim should be to walk briskly; slow walking like sauntering or window shopping is not good and can actually seem to bring on back problems.

Swimming   The chief advantage of swimming is that the water supports the weight of your body while you move around in it. If it is possible to swim three or four times a week on a regular basis, this is ideal.

Swimming is an excellent exercise for most back sufferers as the water holds the weight of the body thus reducing the effects of gravity on the spine, whilst exercising.

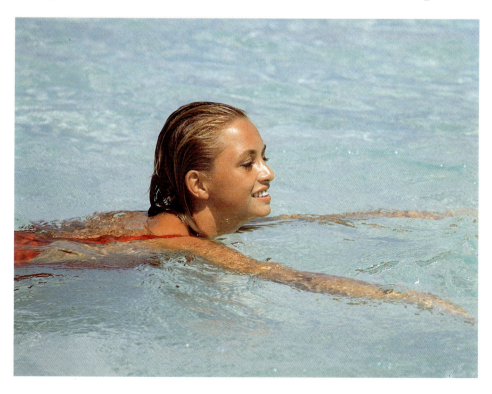

Cycling This activity is excellent exercise for the hips and the knees. They can be exercised without putting any weight on them, and so cycling is especially suitable for people suffering from arthritis in these joints.

Yoga and relaxation Many back sufferers benefit from the gentle exercise of yoga, especially if the patient tends to be a bit stiff. But if the cause of the back problem is loose or hypermobile joints in the spine, then the additional stretch obtained in yoga is not usually beneficial and can actually be harmful. Another advantage of yoga is the relaxation involved, and most people today can benefit from re-learning how to relax. It is ideal for stressed mothers, wives and husbands – whether the stress comes from within the home or from the work environment.

Cycling is a safe sport for most back sufferers; it is also a good aerobic exercise for the heart and lungs.

Other sports Squash, running, jogging, weight training, aerobics and rugby all have their place in an exercise regime. Some sports, however, may not be suitable for particular types of spinal problems, and a chiropractor can usually advise the individual patient on what is safe and what should be avoided.

Squash, for example, is a very aggressive game with many

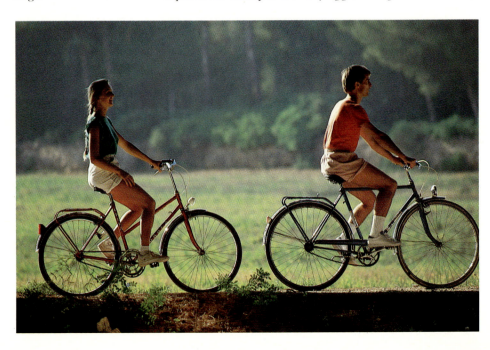

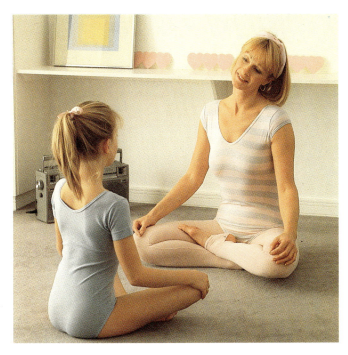

For some people, usually those who suffer from general stiffness and restriction in the back or joints, yoga is a very safe form of exercise, as it is very gentle. The good breathing techniques and relaxation that are part of yoga are also very important.

quick, sharp, movements and low backhands where it is easy to injure the low back and the knees. Squash players also frequently have to stop suddenly and then move off quickly in another direction which again makes them prone to jarring the low back and the knees.

Many rugby players suffer from either low back problems, neck problems, or both. And during the 'aerobics–craze' many would-be exercisers were damaging their ankles, knees, hips and low backs.

At times a chiropractor may need to give specific exercises to a patient to strengthen and tone particular back, abdominal or leg muscles. All these muscles, when toned up, can help to support the spine and make it stronger, and therefore prevent weakness from recurring.

It is not appropriate for a book to describe specific exercises in detail, however, be they stretching type exercises, isometric, isotonic or whatever. This is because each patient has to be advised about exactly the right type of exercise for his or her back problem. The right timing of the start of an exercise programme is also important, and a chiropractor's advice should be sought in each individual case.

CASE HISTORIES

LOW BACK PROBLEMS AFTER PREGNANCY

Mrs E, age 30, consulted the chiropractor with low back pain which had started one week previously after she had fallen and jarred her low back. There was no referred pain down in to either leg.

One year ago she had suffered with some low back pain which was diagnosed by the orthopaedic specialist as being a 'disc problem'. Six to seven weeks ago she noticed some low back discomfort but nothing severe.

She was in excellent general health, having given birth eleven weeks previously.

Examination revealed severe restriction to normal movement in the low back at the level of the fifth lumbar vertebra, and between it and the sacrum on both sides. The rest of the spine had a tendency to restricted movement (hypomobility).

Previous hospital X-rays revealed no abnormality.

The chiropractor diagnosed that the jarring to the low back had caused it to seize up while it was still weak from the recent pregnancy.

Mrs E received manipulative treatment to the low back on both sides and after one treatment she was very much improved. In total, only three treatments were needed in order to solve the low back problem.

PROBLEMS WITH THE YOUNG SPINE

Miss L, age 8, was brought to the chiropractor by her mother. The problem, the mother explained, was that Miss L had difficulty co-ordinating her movements, was hyperactive, immature with a below age reading ability and still wet her bed regularly at night. She had suffered severely as a child with both tonsillitis and mastoiditis and had been born with the umbilical cord round her neck.

The chiropractor then examined the whole spine of Miss L, and found quite a number of severe problems, unusual in a child of her age. There was a severe restriction to the normal movements of the low (lumbar) spine on both sides and a compensatory increase in movement from the third lumbar vertebra upwards on both sides.

There was general tension in the upper back (thoracic region) from the first to the eighth thoracic vertebrae on both sides and tension with restriction in movement of the upper two neck (cervical) vertebrae on both sides. It was also noted that, due to the lower lumbar problems her right leg was slightly shorter than the left.

Due to her age no X-rays were taken. In view of the fact that her spine really needed a 'good service' the chiropractor aimed to restore as much normal movement to the spine as possible, using spinal manipulative therapy.

Four treatments over a two-month period remarkably improved her clarity in thinking and reduced her hyperactivity and frequency in bed wetting.

Over a two-year period Miss L received thirteen treatments in order to maintain her improvement. Most treatments were tied in with holiday periods and so offered no disruption to her normal routine.

FARMER'S BACK

Mr G, a farmer, age 40, consulted the chiropractor with a low back stiffness of one-week duration, accompanied with slight pain down the legs. The problem was aggravated by bending, sneezing, sitting and trying to put on his socks. Relief was obtained with walking and the use of ice-packs on the back.

Mr G had a previous history of low back trouble over the last 20 years which came on initially after stacking and lifting bales of straw. Over the years he had tried both traction and corsets to no avail. In recent years he had successfully used chiropractic treatment for his back pain. His general health was otherwise excellent.

Examination of the spine was extremely painful and restricted in flexion, extension and left side bending. Left straight leg-raising was a positive 80° and movement of the fifth lumbar vertebra was restricted on the left side. X-rays were taken but revealed no abnormalities.

After two treatments, consisting of spinal adjustment, soft-tissue work, ultra-sound and the use of icepacks at home, his problem was completely resolved.

DIY BACK

Mr M, age 45, started with acute low back pain two weeks prior to his visit to the chiropractor. The back pain had started after working in an awkward, twisted position during a DIY weekend. As well as low back pain there was left-leg sciatica.

He had previously suffered with back pain both ten years previously and six months previously. His general health was excellent, but he was overweight, travelled a great deal in his job and ate too many business lunches.

On examination his stance was antalgic, leaning away from the side of the pain. Movements of the back were particularly painful in bending to the side of the pain. The movement of the fifth lumbar vertebra was severely restricted and accompanied by severe muscle spasm.

The chiropractor diagnosed that the likely cause of the problem was due to the fixation of the fifth lumbar vertebra accompanied by strained ligaments between the low back and the ilium (part of the pelvis).

Treatment consisted of soft-tissue muslce work, ultra-sound and spinal adjustments while the patient lay face down. After four treatments he was fully recovered and was advised to wear a weight-lifter's belt when undertaking any further DIY work or gardening. It would be also advantageous for him to lose weight and to take up some regular form of exercise.

LOW BACK PROBLEMS WITH REFERRED PAIN

Mr E, age 45, consulted the chiropractor with acute low back pain with left-leg pain passing to the calf and the toes in the distribution of the nerve root from the fourth lumbar vertebra. The pain had started two to three weeks previously after lifting and he had a past history of back trouble two years and five years previously.

Examination revealed pain and restriction when the patient stretched or bent to the left or right. Movement was restricted in the fourth and fifth lumbar vertebrae and sacrum, but there was excessive movement (hypermobility) from the fourth lumbar vertebra upwards. Knee (patella) and heel (achilles) reflexes were all reduced. There was excessive acute tenderness in the ligaments between the fourth and fifth lumbar vertebrae and the fifth lumbar vertebra and the sacrum. X-rays were taken and showed degenerative changes in the discs and joints of the lumbar spine with narrowing of the spaces where the spinal nerves leave the backbone (intervertebral foramen).

A diagnosis of acute low back strain with ligament damage was made. The severe restriction to normal vertebral movement in the lower lumbar spine would further narrow the intervertebral foramen, thus causing pressure of the spinal nerves leaving the spine in that area. Restoration of normal movement would help to reduce this.

Treatment consisted of appropriate spinal adjustment and the problem was resolved within four treatments.

PROBLEMS WITH MIGRAINE

Mrs J, age 40, consulted the chiropractor for help with chronic migraine headaches which she had suffered with, almost continually, from the age of 16. Mrs J had consulted various doctors and specialists over the years and tried numerous treatments, all to no avail. On the basis of her case history there appeared to be no known cause for her problem.

Examination of Mrs J's spine revealed severe restriction in the normal movement of the vertebrae in the upper part of her neck, across the shoulders and down between the shoulder blades. All neurological tests were normal. General movements of the head and neck were normal. However taking the head backwards and at the same time turning the head from one side to the other produced dizziness.

X-rays showed that the neck was normal except that the two vertebrae at the top of the neck were fused together. In view of this and the examination findings, extreme care needed to be taken when adjusting the top of the neck. However, after four treatments, no change to the symptoms were noted. The chiropractor then examined Mrs J's jaws and found that the jaw joint on the right side was very restricted in movement and the muscles and ligaments around the joint were tender and painful.

The chiropractor then concentrated on treating the jaw joint using soft-tissue massage and manipulation. After one treatment to the jaw Mrs J became completely free from headaches and at the time of writing, many months later, is still headache free.

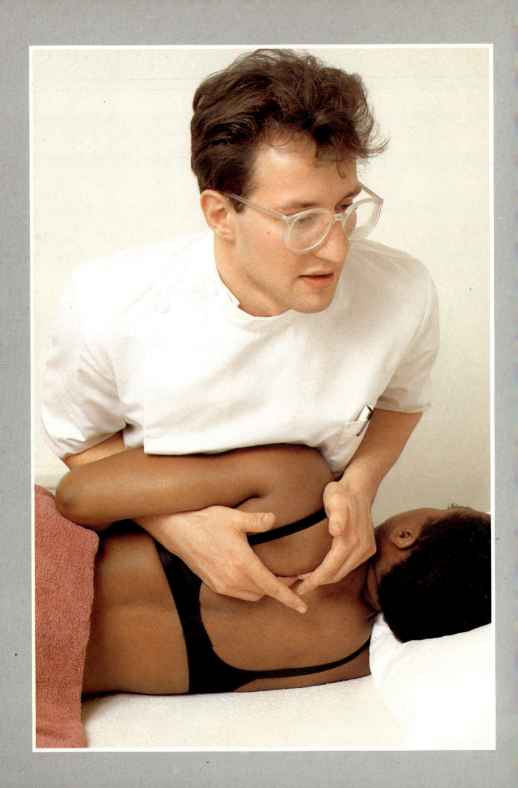

6

RELATED
THERAPIES

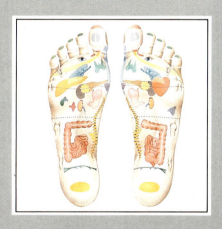

For many conditions, chiropractic treatment may be the only therapy required. But some problems are not that straightforward, and many patients can benefit from an additional or alternative form of treatment. The following are the therapies most commonly used in conjunction with, or as alternatives to, chiropractic.

Chiropractic and massage

Many chiropractors employ some type of massage as part of their overall treatment regime, often before any form of spinal adjustment. There are various kinds of massage, and the type selected is usually the most appropriate to the area that the chiropractor is treating – such as the low back, neck or shoulder. Nearly everyone who regularly receives massage is aware of the tremendous psychological effect it can have. Good massage brings about an overall sense of calm and well-being.

Depending on the severity of the condition, massage may feel relaxing or (in most cases) slightly painful at first, because the chiropractor is trying to relieve muscle spasm and thereby release any stress and tension it has on the spine. During massage, she searches for areas in the muscles that feel

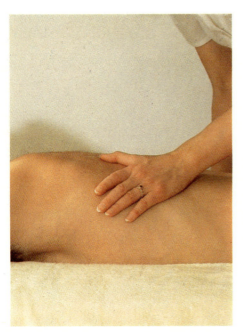
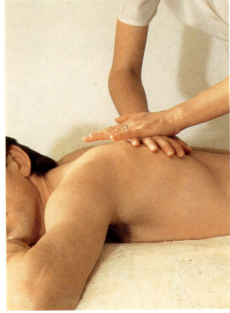

particularly tight or knotted, or have a stringy texture. Usually such locations are quite specific, and can feel particularly tender to the patient. However, by stimulating these 'trigger' points, the chiropractor can bring about an overall relaxation in the muscle concerned. Stimulation of such points increases the circulatory and lymphatic flow in the area, and helps to disperse any toxins that have accumulated there. This in turn reduces the level of any chemical irritants within the muscle itself, and speeds up the healing process.

This type of massage is, of course, quite different from that of the Swedish masseur or beauty therapist. Their techniques are designed specifically to relax, strengthen or stimulate a particular muscle or group of muscles. Chiropractic massage can achieve more than one of these effects at the same time. It also helps to break down any soft-tissue adhesions, and can assist in restoring muscular strength and mobility after an injury.

There are various techniques available to a general masseur, who often uses several of them to achieve the desired combination of muscle relaxation and circulatory stimulation. The four main types are called effleurage, petrissage, friction and tapotement.

These photographs show the four main types of massage used by a masseur/euse: effleurage, petrissage, friction and tapotement. This is quite different to the types of soft-tissue massage used by a chiropractor. There are numerous types of massage techniques used by qualified masseurs. Massage can be either stimulating or relaxing but the overall effect is very beneficial.

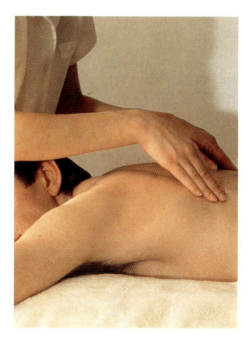

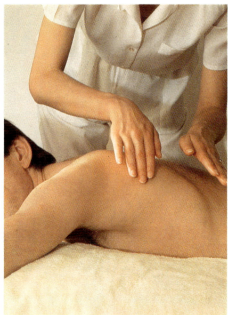

Effleurage consists of long stroking movements to the area being massaged. Its aim is to relax the superficial muscles, and so prepare the way for deeper massage. It is quite soothing, but may at times be applied fairly vigorously to areas with specific muscle tension and knotting.

Petrissage is a type of massage that involves the kneading, rolling and squeezing of muscle tissue, and therefore tends to be a deeper type of massage than effleurage. As a result it is not usually so relaxing, although it certainly achieves its aim of stimulating the tissues concerned.

Friction massage is usually employed specifically to release areas of tension in muscles and to stimulate the circulation. To achieve this, it involves the use of small but deep circular movements, which trap the muscles against the underlying bone to give the massage a more solid base. It is probably the closest to the usual type of chiropractic soft-tissue technique.

Tapotement involves movements such as clapping, cupping and flicking the surface of the skin in order to stimulate and tone up the underlying muscles. This type of massage is frequently used in conjunction with one of the other types.

Massage is therefore often employed before chiropractic treatment for conditions that involve a significant amount of muscle spasm, tension or strain – which can be helped better by a qualified masseur than a chiropractor.

In cases where the cause of a back or neck problem is mainly emotional (because of stress or an inability to relax), an overall relaxing massage is usually of more benefit than a specifically oriented chiropractic treatment. There are probably many other instances in which a good massage immediately before chiropractic adjustment can be beneficial and, because of this, many chiropractors work closely with masseurs – to the overall benefit of their patients.

Chiropractic and Rolfing

Rolfing, otherwise known as structural integration, is a special form of deep massage developed by its originator, Ida Rolf. It is a powerful technique in which the masseur uses his body weight – through the fingers, knuckles and elbows – to loosen the musculature and soften the supporting collagenous fascia of the body. It is a drastic and often painful treatment. Even so it is often extremely effective.

The aim of Rolfing is to loosen and realign the musculature and its support, based on the assumption that the stresses and strains of life impose distortions on the body which become deeply set in the connective tissue. As a result, the shape and contours of the body, as well as its posture, reflect a person's experience and attitudes to life. The masseur (known as a Rolfer) thus aims to correct these distortions by loosening the musculature and allowing it to return to normal – but this is neither a quick nor easy process.

Rolfing is considered as an alternative to chiropractic in cases of severe postural and self-identity problems associated with chronic musculoskeletal pains and tensions. If, following a series of Rolfing treatments, any biomechanical back or neck problems still remain, chiropractic therapy may be used to resolve them.

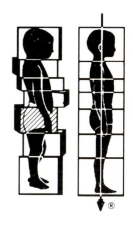

The symbol of Rolfing: Rolfers teach their patients to visualize their bodies as a pile of child's bricks. The aim is to get the tower perpendicular, to realign and reintegrate the parts of the body to make a posturally correct whole.

Chiropractic and aromatherapy

Aromatherapy is a type of massage that employs what are called essential oils, which are derived from natural aromatic essences extracted from wild or cultivated plants. The oils can be used to treat various ailments, because the extracts are thought to have specific healing properties which work on the body when they are absorbed through the skin during massage.

Such oils have been used in similar ways since the time of the Ancient Egyptians. Their expertise with the oils allowed the Egyptians to develop the art of embalming using natural methods. Most of the plant sources have both internal and external applications associated with specific medical conditions. For example, chamomile has been used to treat indigestion, fever, influenza, loss of appetite, insomnia and migraine. Lavender oil can be applied externally for acne, burns, insect bites and wounds. Internally it can be used for conditions such as asthma, coughs, slow digestion and migraine.

In aromatherapy, the oils are used as a massage oil, in conjunction with various massage techniques. The oil is selected according to the type of condition being treated. As a result, aromatherapy can be used in conjunction with certain chiropractic treatments in which massage is indicated. In some cases, aromatherapy alone may be more appropriate, such as when there is chronic muscle tension and strain – whether of physical or emotional origin.

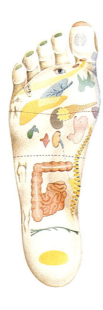

Chiropractic and reflexology

Reflexologists use massage in another way, by massaging specific areas of the feet to bring about an overall change in health. This type of therapy is intended to affect various organs – the different parts of the feet are thought to be related to different parts of the body.

A reflexologist believes that reflexes in the feet are related to all parts of the body, and so massaging a specific area can bring about a reflex change in the organ concerned in the form of either a stimulating or calming effect.

The feet are massaged by the reflexologist with his or her hands – usually the thumbs. The aim is to detect and pin-point certain tender areas. The degree of tenderness depends on how out of balance the corresponding part of the body is. This also, therefore, aids diagnosis. In some of the reflex areas there may be a build-up of the granules, which can be felt by the reflexologist. The granules are believed to be composed of calcium crystals and uric acid, and massage can help to disperse them through the circulatory and excretory systems.

During the massage, both feet are usually treated. Typical

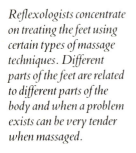

Reflexologists concentrate on treating the feet using certain types of massage techniques. Different parts of the feet are related to different parts of the body and when a problem exists can be very tender when massaged.

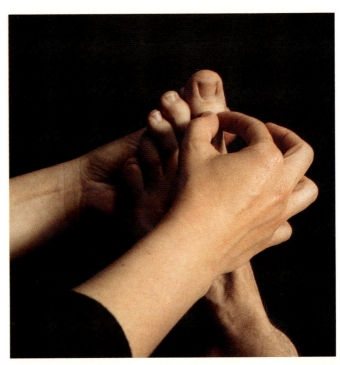

disorders treated in this way include migraine, sinus problems, circulatory disorders, hormonal imbalances, kidney and bladder disorders and symptoms of stress and tension. Sometimes there are reactions to the treatment in the form of a healing crisis before healing proper commences. There are also a number of conditions that should not be treated by reflexology, and for this reason it is essential to seek the advice of a qualified practitioner.

Ultimately the aim of the reflexologist is to disperse the waste deposits (granules) from the feet, reduce congestion and remove any blockages to the energy pathways of the body (as in the theory that underlies acupuncture). The effect is to balance the body's polarity (energy flow), improve the circulation and normalize the functions of organs and glands. Overall the treatment has a relaxing effect and brings about a feeling of well-being.

Reflexology is seldom used in conjunction with chiropractic, although it is probably true to say that many chiropractic patients can benefit from the cumulative effects of reflexology. The chiropractor may refer the patient when suitable.

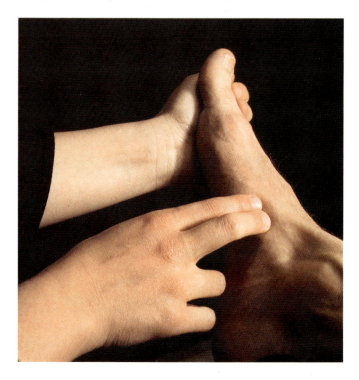

Chiropractic and the Alexander technique

If you see somebody with a superb posture, who appears to glide when he or she walks and who sits upright at all times, you are probably observing a person who is a practitioner of the Alexander technique. The method is especially popular with professional musicians, actors, singers and dancers, who many years ago realized the benefits of this particular approach to promoting good health.

The aim of an Alexander teacher is to detect postural faults and ways in which a person misuses his or her body, and to give guidance about how to correct such faults. From an early age, we tend to develop habits of postural misuse that can result in a wide range of effects – particularly problems such as backache, headaches and neck pain. Loss of voice production, breathing problems and general tension can all result from bad posture.

In fact very few people these days have a good posture, and so most of us can benefit from the Alexander technique. The teacher identifies aspects of poor posture and shows the person how to reuse the body properly. This usually starts with learning to sit, stand and lie properly, and then progresses to walking and the general use of the body in everyday life in such a manner as to minimize stresses.

It is not easy to re-learn how to use your body in this way, and it can take many months or years to perfect, but in the end it is well worth the effort. Any chiropractic patient with a posture problem can benefit from the Alexander technique. One difficulty, however, is that Alexander teachers are few in number and so are not widely available.

Chiropractic and osteopathy

The relationship between chiropractic and osteopathy has been considered in chapter 3, *Chiropractic in context*. Osteopathy practised in the United States also encompasses the use of drugs and surgery and is therefore not representative of the technique as it is practised generally in Britain. The latter, more fundamental form is considered here, because the essential principles remain common to both, while their combination with orthodox medical techniques in the United States adds nothing to our understanding of the alternative science.

Osteopaths treat a wide variety of musculoskeletal disorders and their effects on the internal organs, using soft-tissue techniques, mobilization and manipulation. However, research has yet to tell us which treatment is more effective for a

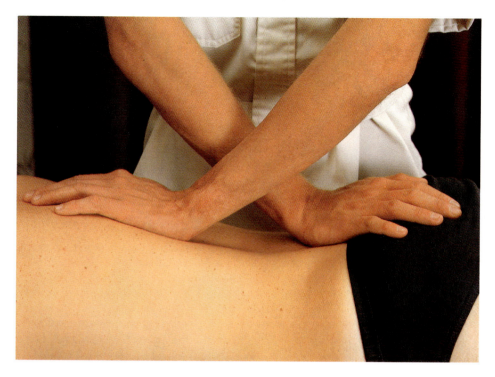

given type of condition. In any case this would be extremely difficult, because an individual practitioner's techniques can vary a great deal, and some have a particular liking for treating specific types of problems for which they find themselves more effective. At the present time, most patients consult a chiropractor or an osteopath on personal recommendation from a satisfied customer. Some patients attend both for treatment, and find one practitioner to be more effective than the other. Thus it tends to be a matter of individual choice or availability that determines which type of practitioner a patient consults.

The osteopath will use different types of mobilization and manipulative techniques to those used by the chiropractor.

Chiropractic and acupuncture

Acupuncture is a separate system of medicine that is complete in itself, rather than being complementary to orthodox medicine. It involves stimulation of points on defined lines that run through the body, characteristically by the insertion of very fine needles into the skin. These so-called acupuncture points are related to the lines called energy meridians that run throughout the body. The course of the meridians and the

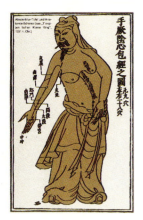

Two of the meridian lines (pathways) of what the Chinese term the body's energy or 'Qi'. Acupuncture treats a person at points along these lines to restore healing harmony and balance to the system.

points on them all have specific locations, which an acupuncturist is able to detect.

An acupuncturist uses the case history and symptoms of the patient to try to determine which system of the body is not functioning correctly. He or she asks various questions, which may appear to be unassociated with the person's complaint – for example, all about his or her childhood, likes and dislikes, dreams and emotions, as well as more normal questions concerning the body, such as the functioning of the stomach, bowels and bladder. The acupuncturist is able to respond to the body 'smell' and the colour of the face and may also examine the eyes, nails, tongue, skin, hair and ears.

The acupuncturist also checks the six pulses he or she can rdetect in each wrist, which are related to a different lines or meridians within the body – and therefore with different systems such as the respiratory, circulatory or digestive system.

These and other tests enable the acupuncturist to locate the system that is in imbalance and does not function properly, and could therefore be the cause of the symptoms the patient is exhibiting. Sometimes more than one system may be at fault, or one system may affect another; some systems may be sluggish, others overactive. For these reasons, acupuncture is an extremely complicated diagnostic tool.

Once a diagnosis has been made, however, the acupuncturist uses fine needles or other stimulation of the acupuncture points to bring about a change in the body. Sometimes the needles are put straight in and straight out, sometimes they are left in and moved gently, and sometimes they are accompanied by moxibustion – the burning of the herb mugwort at the outer ends of the needles.

Some chiropractors and osteopaths use acupuncture in association with their manipulative techniques. Most, however, refer a patient to an acupuncturist when they think it necessary, usually for problems that require an overall system of medicine. Such conditions include digestive upsets, kidney and bladder disorders, problems with menstrual periods, general lack of energy, insomnia and depression.

Someone suffering with chronic arthritis throughout the body might benefit more from a system of treatment such as acupuncture than from chiropractic treatment. In some cases, what appears at first to be a straightforward biomechanical back problem does not respond to chiropractic treatment, but does to acupuncture. But nobody, as yet, fully understands why.

Chiropractic and medical herbalism

Medical herbalism is another complete system of medicine. It is the treatment of disease using medicinal plants, either internally or externally, to restore the health of the patient. It is therefore a natural method of healing, based on the traditional use of herbs coupled with today's scientific knowledge.

Before the onset of modern medicine, many people in various parts of the world relied on herbs to cure sickness and disease, a system of treatment that dates back before recorded history. It is only in the last hundred years or so that herbalism has been overtaken by modern methods and drugs – but even some of today's medicinal drugs, such as aspirin (a derivative of willow bark) and digitalis (from foxgloves), have their origins in herbal medicine.

Like an acupuncturist, a herbalist frequently treats the person and not the symptom, and may spend a considerable time on the patient's general history. Like acupuncture, herbalism can treat a wide variety of conditions, such as colds etc., bronchitis, eczema, asthma, gastric problems, bowel problems, cystitis, kidney disorders, headaches, arthritis, fevers and infections, migraine, heart and circulatory disorders, ulcers, gynaecological conditions and hormonal problems. The different herbal remedies are not necessarily specific

A fanciful view of a physic garden from the 16th-century herbal Den Groten Herbarius. *The garden was in effect the laboratory and pharmacy of the herbalist, where the raw materials for herbal medicine were grown.*

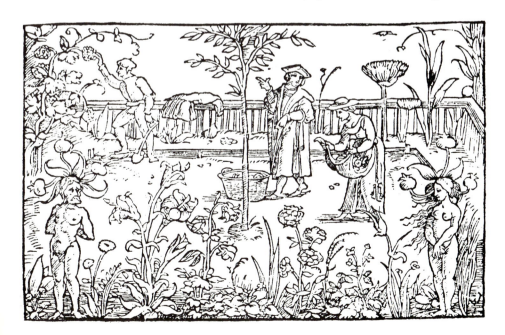

to a condition but may be used to treat the whole person.

Medicinal herbs can have many actions. They can relax organs and tissues, stimulate, astringe or sedate, eliminate toxins and waste products, and help to overcome the effects of infections, enhance the circulation, aid appetite and digestion, and reduce irritation and inflammation, and regulate the secretion of hormones.

Herbal remedies can be prescribed in various forms, but the most common is a tincture. This is a concentrated extract of herbs mixed with water and alcohol. Herbal infusions are also frequently given, and prepared in much the same way as a pot of tea. And some herbal remedies are made up as tablets.

As with acupuncture, many chiropractic patients have conditions that can benefit from treatment by a herbalist. But apart from conditions such as digestive upsets, kidney and bladder disorders, gynaecological problems and PMS (premenstrual syndrome), the most likely reason for a chiropractor to recommend herbalism would be in the case of a patient suffering with severe arthritis throughout the body, for which chiropractic manipulation would not be a suitable choice of therapy.

Chiropractic and homeopathy

Homeopathy is similar to acupuncture and herbalism, in that it is another complete system of treatment, in which the practitioner is more concerned with the person as a whole than with individual symptoms. A homeopath therefore prescribes remedies with this approach in mind.

Homeopathic remedies may be animal, vegetable or mineral in origin. Sometimes herbal remedies are used, as well as extracts from certain drugs such as morphine and cocaine.

Homeopathy is based on the principle of treating like with like. For example, if it is known that a certain remedy causes a certain effect in a healthy person – such as a red itchy rash – then a patient exhibiting this symptom may be treated with that same remedy. This is because homeopaths believe symptoms are the signs of the body's fight against a disease and that by encouraging the symptons the body's fight becomes more effective. As with the other therapies, it takes a considerable time to investigate a patient as a whole, rather than an individual symptom, before the practitioner can prescribe the ideal individual remedy or remedies.

In order to avoid unwanted side-effects, homeopaths have developed a system in which they prescribe the smallest effective dose that will bring about a return to health. To accomplish this, the remedies are diluted many times, a process known as potentization. It is believed that in general the greater the dilution, the greater is the effect of the remedy.

Again, a chiropractor may refer patients with various problems to a homeopath, for conditions that would not normally be suitable for chiropractic treatment. But, as with the other therapies, certain conditions such as headache, migraine, backache, or arthritis may respond better to homeopathy than to chiropractic manipulation.

Chiropractic and physiotherapy

There are many medical establishments throughout the world in which chiropractors and physiotherapists work side by side, the treatment given by one complementing that of the other.

A chiropractor is a specialist in spinal and joint manipulation, with some associated soft-tissue techniques. A physiotherapist, on the other hand, uses many techniques with which a chiropractor is not well acquainted. These include the use of machines such as ultra-sound, diathermy, interferential and short-wave, and various mobilization techniques, exercises and massage regimes. Thus the two professions should be able to work well together for the overall benefit of a patient, rather than to compete in the narrow field of manipulation. This is certainly so for back, spinal and joint-related conditions.

Chiropractic and applied kinesiology

Applied kinesiology is a technique that was developed by a chiropractor, and it can be used as a system of diagnosis and treatment for a variety of conditions, in addition to back and joint problems. The method detects incorrect joint function, spinal lesions, muscle weakness and organic dysfunction. These are discovered by testing relative muscle strength – usually resulting in the location of a weak muscle. Various individual muscles have been related to different organ systems within the body, and each muscle has reflex and trigger points that can be stimulated in order to bring about a return to normal, either within the organ or in the skeletal system.

Some chiropractors use this type of testing as an aid to localize and treat a particular spinal problem. Some have developed applied kinesiology to such an extent that they use it as an alternative to spinal manipulation. It should be pointed out, however, that not all chiropractors actively practise this technique.

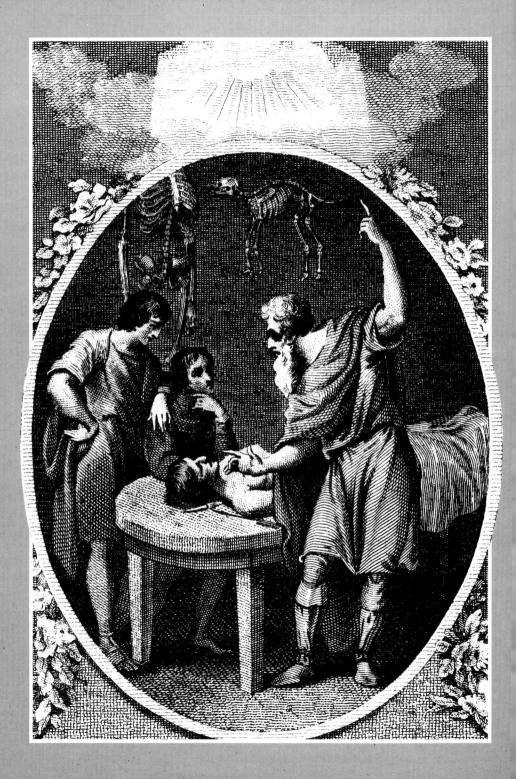

7

FOUNDATIONS
OF CHIROPRACTIC

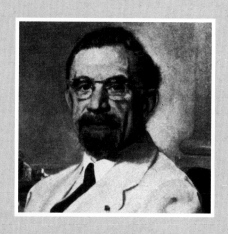

Chiropractic was founded by Daniel David Palmer (1845-1913). He was born in the Canadian backwoods, and as a young boy was always taking home injured animals to 'heal'. He spent much of his adolescence reading books on the anatomy and functioning of the human body. During his early adult life he dabbled in various jobs: he was an itinerant trader, he taught at school and he managed to make and lose a number of mercantile fortunes in Illinois and Iowa in the United States. In 1886 he finally settled in Burlington, Iowa, where he practised for nine years as a magnetic healer.

Although Palmer was not medically qualified, most authors agree that he was an intelligent man who had the knack of healing. His interest in magnetic healing was aroused when he met an internationally famous therapist of this type called Paul Caster, who was also from Burlington. And it was during this time in Burlington that Palmer continued to develop his interest in the spine and how it functions, eventually concluding that misaligned vertebrae might well be a primary cause of disease. From this his theory that structure governs function probably arose.

In 1895 he had an office in the Putnam Building, Davenport, Iowa. One day the janitor of the building, Harvey Lillard, told Palmer how he had become almost completely deaf seventeen years previously after he had heard something go crack in his neck. This had happened while Lillard was exerting himself in a cramped and awkward position. Because of his interest in the spine, Palmer examined Lillard and found that one of his vertebrae was out of position. Palmer persuaded Lillard to allow him to try to correct the malposition and, so the story goes, after adjustments on three consecutive days Lillard's hearing returned.

There is some historical confusion as to whether the vertebra involved was the fourth thoracic vertebra (in the upper back) or the second cervical vertebra (in the neck). Palmer's son, B J Palmer, attested to the latter and said that he watched the adjustments being done, although it has to be said that at the time when Palmer was effecting Lillard's 'cure' his son was only about fourteen years old.

Contemporary members of the medical profession were naturally sceptical that a man's hearing could have been restored in this way, believing that it was scientifically impossible. Lillard's own doctor, however, confirmed the previous deafness and the restoration of his hearing.

Following this 'miraculous' occurrence, Palmer then

attempted to treat a patient with an 'untreatable' heart complaint by adjusting the spine. In a similar manner the patient responded to the adjustment and immediate relief was obtained.

D D Palmer was not discouraged by the sceptics – in fact he was inclined to regard their reaction as a challenge. He set out to further increase his knowledge about the structure and function of the spine from the medical information then available. He also made a detailed study of the nervous system. Armed with this knowledge, he then went on to develop a therapeutic technique of spinal adjustment, which he promoted with an evangelical fervour wherever he went. This type of enthusiasm for anything new was also typical of the United States at that time.

In 1896 Palmer began his first school on the fourth floor of the Ryan Building (as the Putnam Building was then renamed), known as Dr Palmer's School and Cure. Later the name of the school was changed to the Palmer Institute and Chiropractic Infirmary.

The orthodox medical profession continued its virulent opposition to both the school and its teachings, however. As a result, Palmer was convicted of practising medicine without a licence and jailed for his sins. He was the first to be convicted, but many others followed. This opposition only reinforced the determination of the early chiropractors to establish the validity of their profession. Although their persistence was admirable, and we can be thankful for it today, to some extent the intense medical opposition was understandable too. After all, the chiropractors were attracting patients away from the doctors, they made claims the orthodox practitioners felt were unjustified, and they advertised their services. This brought them to the attention of the public and the medical opposition. (Medical doctors were allowed to advertise before 1910, but the better class of physician did not care to do it.)

By 1902 fifteen graduates had passed through the school, including Palmer's son, B J Palmer, who was still only 21 years old. A few years later D D Palmer left the school in the hands of his son and went to spread the word about chiropractic throughout the Indian Territory, California and Oregon. He founded a museum for the collection of osteological specimens and by 1928 this was declared 'without doubt, the best collection of human spines in existence' by an investigation team from the Council on Medical Education and Hospitals, a committee of the American Medical Association.

Countries with chiropractic legislation:
- Australia
- Canada
- Guam
- Liechtenstein
- Namibia
- Norway
- New Zealand
- Panama
- Puerto Rico
- South Africa
- Switzerland
- United Arab Emirates
- USA
- Virgin Island
- Yugoslavia
- Zimbabwe

Countries where chiropractic is legal under common law:
- Bermuda
- Denmark
- Great Britain
- The Netherlands
- Sweden

In 1913 he returned to Davenport, Iowa, where he was accidentally run down by a car driven by his son. D D Palmer then left Davenport again and went to Los Angeles where, three months later, he died. There is no indication that his death was a consequence of the car accident.

The background to chiropractic

In the nineteenth century many physicians and surgeons documented the relationship between the nervous system, spinal disorders and ill health. These investigators were forerunners of much of the medical knowledge we have built on today.

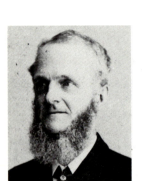

Thomas Pridgin Teale FRCS 1801-1867.

Among them, one who was particularly interesting from a chiropractic point of view was the Englishman, Thomas Pridgin Teale, who was a Fellow of the Royal College of Surgeons and of the Royal Society. When the Medical Act was passed in 1858 he was one of the six nominees of the Crown for a seat in the Medical Council. Among his researches, he identified areas of referred pain or neuralgia associated with the cervical, thoracic and lumbar areas of the spine. He also related symptoms such as dyspepsia, flatulence, heartburn and breathing problems to tenderness in certain areas of the spine.

Although he was an outstanding figure in many ways, Teale was not alone in his interest in such investigations, which were being pursued also in America, France and Germany, despite the fact that the main thrust of medical treatment still consisted of applying leeches, purgatives and ointments to cure most ills.

It would be a mistake, however, to think that spinal manipulation itself was invented in the nineteenth century. There is abundant evidence that it has been practised for centuries in some form or other – although almost certainly not as part of an integrated therapeutic system prior to this time. Historical references trace the art of manipulation back to Hippocrates (460-377 BC) and even to China some two thousand years before that.

Archaic antecedents

The use of manipulation in healing has been described in ancient Chinese texts dating from 2700 BC, by the Greeks in 1500 BC, and by the Early Egyptians, who documented its use in the treatment of sprained, displaced, dislocated and even crushed vertebrae.

Hippocrates was the first physician to identify a link between spinal problems and ill health, and he is also known to have developed a table for guidance in treating spinal problems. The Greek physician Claudius Galen (AD130-200), a celebrated medical writer and anatomist who attained great fame while living in Rome and whose reputation dominated medicine during the early Roman Empire, was the first to emphasize the overall importance of the nervous system. It was Galen who discovered the existence of spinal nerves and defined three different regions of the spine, the cervical, thoracic and lumbar areas.

During the Middle Ages, after a long period of neglect, spinal manipulation became popular again. It was part of the practice of 'bone setting', and bone-setters, as the practitioners of this unsophisticated yet frequently effective skill are known, still exist in some parts of the world even today. Most were unschooled by modern standards, and learned their craft as a tradition of techniques that were handed down from adult to child, commonly from father to son. In medieval times bone-setters were often renowned as gifted healers who could

A slight case of overmanning? This is how the ancient Greeks dealt with a dislocated shoulder.

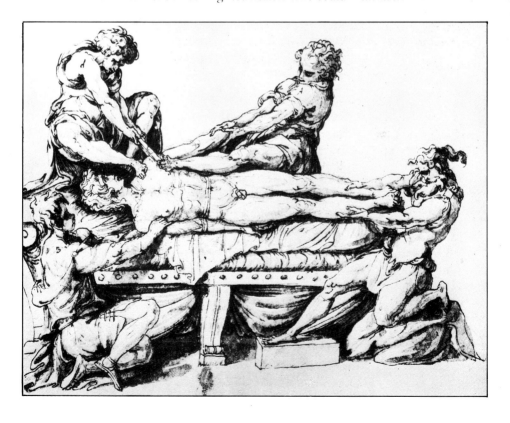

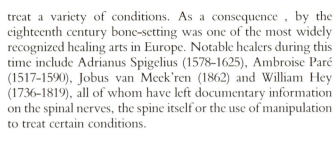

treat a variety of conditions. As a consequence , by the eighteenth century bone-setting was one of the most widely recognized healing arts in Europe. Notable healers during this time include Adrianus Spigelius (1578-1625), Ambroise Paré (1517-1590), Jobus van Meek'ren (1862) and William Hey (1736-1819), all of whom have left documentary information on the spinal nerves, the spine itself or the use of manipulation to treat certain conditions.

B J Palmer (1881-1961)

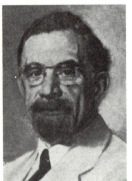

B J Palmer 1881-1961.

When Bartlett Joshua Palmer took over his father's fledgling school he was only 25 years of age. The father may have been the founder of chiropractic, but it was left to the son to develop it and establish a firm basis for the continuation of the profession to the present day. By the time he died in 1961, he had developed chiropractic into the second largest health care system in the United States, in spite of continuing opposition from the medical profession.

During his lifetime B J Palmer established himself as the prophet of chiropractic, with Davenport as its Mecca. He has been described as a genius with a brilliant organizational mind who was not only a teacher and lecturer but also a prolific author and pioneer radio and television broadcaster. He wrote 30 books, edited two of the earliest chiropractic publications, and contributed thousands of hours to radio and television. In his younger days he was a striking figure with flowing black hair. He was usually seen in a white linen suit with a long black silk bow tie – a man who certainly intended to make his mark.

B J Palmer also installed a printing press at the school, which each year produced millions of tracts on chiropractic. He established a research clinic in 1935, and took over a facility for mental patients – Clear View Sanitarium – where senior students could observe and practise.

For two decades, until 1924, B J Palmer was the undisputed leader of chiropractic. But from 1924 until his death in 1961 he was really leader in name only. The reason for this, ironically, lay in one of his own inventions. In 1924, at the annual PSC lyceum, an assembly of some 4000 chiropractors, B J introduced a heat-sensitive instrument which he called the neurocalometer. He claimed that this instrument was able to locate subluxations in the spine as a result of detecting rises in temperature on the surface of the skin, and at the meeting declared that no chiropractor could properly practise without one of the instruments. The consequence of this claim – or

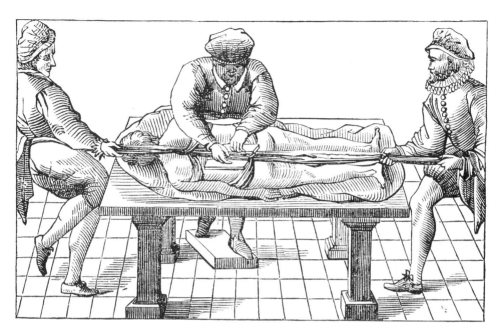

perhaps of the force with which it was made – was that a massive wave of purists, chiropractors who used their hands only, defected from B J and his teachings.

He came into further conflict with other members of the profession because he felt that many of them were starting to follow the osteopathic route. Today he would be amazed to see just how the profession has developed throughout the world and no doubt proud to see that it has remained such a valuable source of primary health care.

Willard Carver

The third famous name in the development of chiropractic was Willard Carver, who was born in 1876. He was a lawyer by profession and practised law in Iowa for fourteen years. His specialization in claims for injuries sustained through employers' negligence necessitated a good working knowledge of anatomy and physiology and this drew him towards the new healing science that was developing in his home state.

He studied chiropractic initially under D D Palmer, but believed that chiropractors should supplement their treatment with the use of adjuncts such as heat, diet and psychotherapy. As a result he was involved in a philosophical debate with the Palmers which stretched over four decades.

Spinal adjustment in the 16th century appears to have been a strenuous undertaking for both patient and practitioner. This was the method favoured by Ambrose Paré (1517-1590), the French physician acknowledged as the father of modern surgery. He believed that distortion of the spine was caused by dislocated vertebrae. The Paré method of relocating vertebrae involved stretching the spine by pulling on towels wrapped tightly round the patient, forcing the vertebrae into place, and splinting them in position for as long as necessary.

Willard Carver spread his teachings of chiropractic in the Indian Territory and started a chiropractic school in Oklahoma City. At one time he presided over four different schools in different states, which granted doctorates not only in chiropractic, but also in philosophy.

Reverend Samuel Weed

Samuel Weed was one of D D Palmer's most devoted patients and he coined the name chiropractic, coming from the two Greek words *cheiro* and *praktikos*, meaning 'to be done by hand'. Unfortunately, today the word has little immediate meaning because few people are familiar with Greek nowadays, but despite this the term has stood the test of time.

The use of X-rays by chiropractors

X-rays were discovered by Wilhelm Röntgen in Würzburg, Germany, in 1895. They were so named because they were of unknown origin, but their development revolutionized medical thinking. Chiropractors were among the first therapists to appreciate the value of X-rays and to utilize them regularly for studying the spine.

With his other achievements, B J Palmer established X-ray laboratories at his school and in 1908 these were among the first and finest in any healing institution – just thirteen years after Röntgen's discovery. In 1910 the Palmer School of Chiropractic in Davenport, Iowa, had courses available in X-ray studies and was the first to use extensive X-rays to detect spinal misalignments.

During World War I, rapid progress was made in the development of X-rays in the United States. By 1918 the Universal College of Chiropractic in Pittsburgh, Pennsylvania, produced the first X-ray photographs of the spine taken with the patient in an upright, standing position. In 1932 Dr Warren L Sausser, who was a chiropractor in New York, produced the first full-length single exposure X-ray of the entire spine.

The chiropractic profession in both the United States and Europe has continued to pioneer the taking of moving X-ray pictures of the spinal column and they still see the use of X-rays as an important diagnostic tool today.

The development of chiropractic training

Before World War I, numerous chiropractic schools opened across the United States, some of which were in the same

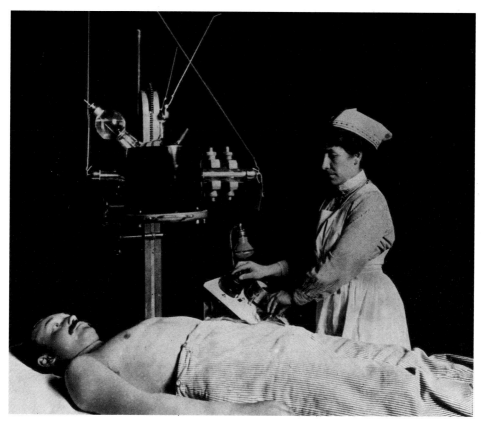

category as the many medical schools that were forced to close in the first two decades of this century. With little in the way of equipment and facilities, many were essentially for-profit institutions and 'diploma mills'. Of the few legitimate institutions founded in that period, some have survived such as the Palmer College (1896), the National College (1906), the Los Angeles College (1911), the Western States College (1906), the Texas College (1908) and the Cleveland College in Los Angeles (1908). The American School in Cedar Rapids, Iowa was a significant early school as was the Universal College and Carver College, both of which merged into existing institutions today. Two unaccredited schools (Sherman and Pennsylvania 'Straight') are now talking with the Council for Chiropractic Education, the government recognized body for chiropractic education in the USA.

During the period 1920 to 1960, several chiropractic

Chiropractic and X-ray technology developed almost contemporarily. Wilhelm Röntgen discovered X-rays in 1895, and by 1908 B J Palmer had not only grasped their significance and potential as a diagnostic tool for chiropractic, but had established X-ray laboratories at his school in Davenport, Iowa.

hospitals and sanitariums were opened in the United States, but frequently they lasted only as long as their benefactor's financial backing. The schools did manage to survive, however, and today in the United States there are fifteen colleges of chiropractic, nationwide, which are recognized by the US Council for Chiropractic Education (CCE). The CCE and its Commission on Accreditation are recognized by the Commissioner of Education in the US Department of Education and the Council on Postsecondary Accreditation.

'Straights' versus 'Mixers'

From the early days in the development of chiropractic there were divergent schools of thought, and these became known as the 'straights' and the 'mixers'. The 'straights' were purists, chiropractors who relied on spinal manipulation as their therapeutic tool. The 'mixers' on the other hand wanted to incorporate a wide range of healing methods within their scope, particularly naturopathy, but also physiotherapy, hydrotherapy and exercise. As early as the 1920s some schools even pressed for the inclusion of minor surgery, obstetrics, optometry and general hospital work in their curriculum. As a result the various schools tended to develop different approaches, depending on the beliefs of their founders.

Because of the two points of view, the United States saw the development of two different chiropractic associations to represent the two groups and to protect their different ideals and interests. These were the International Chiropractors Association (ICA), which represented the 'straights', and the American Chiropractic Association (ACA), which represented the 'mixers'. The two organizations have remained separate to the present day, although their differences are probably not so great as they used to be. Only about 10–15 per cent might be 'straight'.

In 1987 the two associations started to discuss the possibility of unifying the chiropractic profession in the United States without either group losing its sense of freedom or differences in philosophy.

European chiropractors

The development of chiropractic in Europe is not so well documented as in the USA, but it is believed to have been introduced to Britain by graduates of the Palmer School in about 1908. The British Chiropractic Association was founded in 1925, and this was followed some years later by the formation of a European Chiropractic Union.

For the most part, chiropractic in Europe gravitated towards the 'straight' beliefs, with more unification than division among the profession throughout the continent. The most controversial subject in Europe arose during the 1930s over B J Palmers 'hole in one' (HIO) theory. His idea was to bring chiropractors back to the 'straight' philosophy – that is, to adjusting the spine, particularly the upper cervical area, exclusively. Following a meeting in London in 1934 which B J Palmer addressed, the differences between the HIOers and the non-HIOers threatened to split the profession. At this stage some chiropractors of the 'mixer' variety, and thus non-HIOers, joined a nature cure association as nature healers rather than as chiropractors. Thus the 'mixers' found their niche in Britain among the nature cure movement.

Today in Europe, there is no apparent segregation into 'straights' and 'mixers'; each individual chiropractor is able to develop and follow his own particular interest. However, the mainstay of chiropractic treatment must still be in the science and art of manipulation, and any other treatment is seen merely as an adjunct.

The growth of chiropractic
From its humble beginnings less than a hundred years ago, chiropractic has developed into the second largest primary health care profession in the world – numbering in the region of 45,000 practitioners worldwide. This also makes chiropractic the largest manipulative profession in the world.

While chiropractic was spreading through the United States in the early twentieth century, it was also moving into Canada, Europe and Australia. Today chiropractors can be found in most countries outside of the Soviet Bloc and China, although in some countries the numbers are extremely small.

Chiropractic was first licensed in the United States in Kansas in 1913. By 1963 New York became the 47th state to license chiropractors, followed by Massachusetts in 1966. All 50 states now grant licences to chiropractors, and graduates of recognized chiropractic colleges are eligible to sit the state licensing examinations. Many, if not most, states recognize other state boards, and through the National Board of Chiropractic Examiners (NBCE) provide for licensing in several states at once through national examinations.

The practice of chiropractic in Canada is governed by legislation that varies from province to province. The first province to bring in Provincial Acts covering chiropractic was Ontario in 1925, followed soon after by Newfoundland. The Canadian Chiropractic Association is the only one in Canada and was federally chartered in 1953. At the present time there are about 3,000 qualified chiropractors in Canada.

Chiropractic was introduced to Australia just after World War I, and the Australian Chiropractors' Association (ACA) was formed in 1938 to represent a mere 22 practitioners in the country. Growth of the profession was exceedingly slow, and twenty years later membership still numbered only 55.

Between 1960 and 1980 the number of chiropractic schools grew in Australia, but some included treatment by naturopathic and osteopathic techniques in their courses. As a result there was a great difference in the philosophies of American-trained and Australian-trained chiropractors, and a second association – the United Chiropractors Association – was formed.

In more recent years the number of Australian colleges has dwindled to two: the Phillip Institute of Technology/School of Chiropractic in Melbourne and the Sydney College of Chiropractic. The two chiropractic associations still exist, representing about 1,500 chiropractors between them, and the organizations work closely together. The first legislation to register chiropractors was in 1964, and today licensure and registration requirements tend to vary from state to state.

In Europe, The Anglo European College of Chiropractic started in 1965 to train European Chiropractors and more recently a new French Chiropractic College has opened in Paris. Switzerland is the only country with complete legislation for chiropractic. The first chiropractors went to Switzerland in the early 1900s, and the first of the 26 cantons to pass a chiropractic law was Lucerne in 1937; the last was Berne in 1974.

Throughout the rest of Europe chiropractors tend to practise under the provisions of common law or Napoleonic law. In many of the countries the chiropractic professions are continually urging their governments to follow the lead of others in requiring licensure for the profession.

Chiropractic today
In common with other health professions throughout the world, chiropractic has a standardized form of training which can be obtained at recognized training colleges in various countries. This means that a qualified chiropractor from

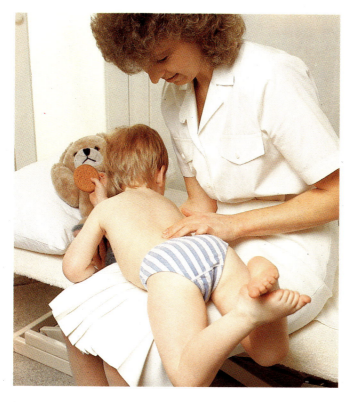

Small children sometimes need reassurance before chiropractic treatment, but most chiropractors are used to putting them at ease.

Britain or the United States can visit most countries and find another qualified chiropractor practising in a similar manner, with similar beliefs and philosophies.

In common with other professions, this gives chiropractors a feeling of unity and parity, wherever in the world they may meet. Coupled with this are the disputes (often with the orthodox medical profession) that many chiropractors have had during their careers. Indeed many of them are still fighting today in order to maintain their place in the overall health care systems in various countries around the world.

Such opposition has not inhibited the development or diminished the numbers of chiropractors. History shows that they are sincere in their beliefs and will continue to practice against all odds. Some ask: why do they do this? The reason is simple – they have the utmost faith in the therapy they are using, based not only on their own experience but also on sound scientific knowledge which they utilize for the good of their patients in bringing about relief from pain and suffering

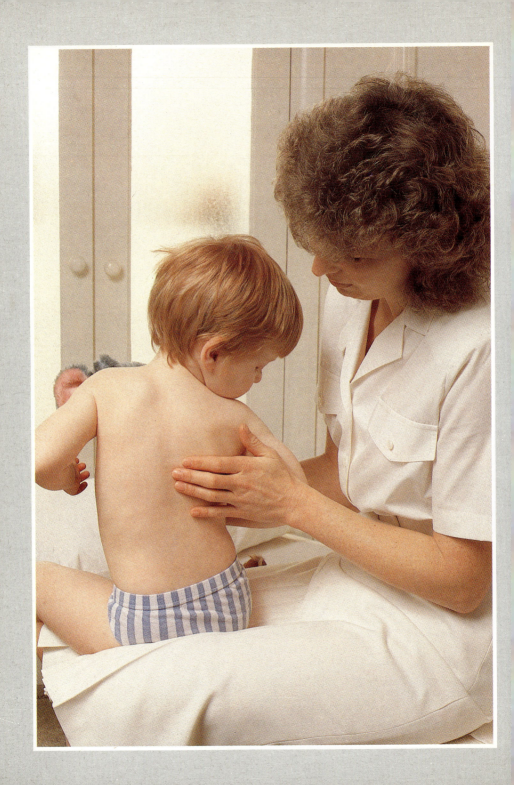

8

FINDING AND CONSULTING A CHIROPRACTOR

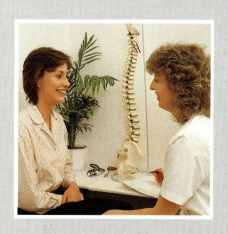

If you decide that chiropractic could help you or your family it is essential to make sure that you choose a qualified chiropractor.

This is not as easy to do as finding an orthodox medical practitioner because at the moment anyone can set up in consulting rooms and call themselves a chiropractor and remain within the law.

The law as it affects chiropractic varies around the world. In the UK and most of Europe (except in Switzerland and Leichtenstein) there is no legislation that protects the use of the word chiropractor, although of course the common law of the country applies.

In the United states, Canada, Australia, New Zealand and some other countries there is legislation which is specific to chiropractic. In the USA this varies from state to state. The malpractice laws which protect the public from mistakes made by orthodox medical doctors also apply to chiropractic, although these rarely need to be implemented.

So if the law is a bit of a minefield how can you be sure that the chiropractor you choose is properly qualified?

The only way you can make sure a chiropractor is fully qualified is to check that they belong to a national chiropractic association. Membership confirms that a practitioner has completed the necessary training course and that as members of a professional organization, they are bound by its code of ethics and discipline which protects you as a patient.

Such associations exist worldwide and each usually has a register of members which is available to the public. In Europe, each member of the appropriate national association automatically becomes a member of the European Chiropractors' Union, which also issues a register of all its members. (See addresses.)

In the United States there are two such associations, the American Chiropractic Association in Virginia with 20,000 members, and the International Chiropractors' Association in Washington DC with about 8500 members. These two associations are currently discussing a merger. At the moment, it is probably better to contact both for a list of qualified chiropractors in your state.

The education of a chiropractor

The training of qualified chiropractors is now standardized throughout the world, and consists of a four-year full-time course at a recognized college. These courses include all the necessary basic science subjects, as with a medical course, and offer training in a cross-section of chiropractic manipulative techniques. Worldwide there are a number of colleges, recognized by the various national associations. Currently there are fifteen colleges in the United States, two in Australia, and one each in Britain, Canada and France.

Graduates of the various colleges are eligible to join the national associations. In some countries, before a graduate is able to practise, he or she has to undertake further registration or pass licensing examinations; this is the case in the United states, Australia and Canada.

How to find a chiropractor

Most of a chiropractor's new patients consult the chiropractor on the personal recommendation of an existing patient. Some patients read about chiropractic or hear it mentioned on the radio, and write to the national association for general information on the subject. The national associations will also, on request, supply the name, address and telephone number of the nearest chiropractic clinic.

In the UK chiropractors are allowed limited advertising and of course they may be listed in a directory such as the Yellow Pages. In the United States advertising is allowed, and some chiropractors do use this method. On the whole, however, American chiropractors prefer not to advertise.

Making an appointment to consult a chiropractor

Once you know the address and telephone number of a clinic and want to make an appointment, you simply telephone the clinic. The clinic secretary or receptionist who answers the telephone will help you to make an appointment to see the chiropractor. The waiting time for a consultation can vary from a day or so to a week or two. Chiropractors tend to be busy people; their services are often in great demand and so it is unusual, unless they have a cancellation, for you to be fitted in immediately, unless you are a really urgent case.

Often prospective patients are referred by their friends or neighbours to a particular chiropractor in a clinic and, if you request a certain named chiropractor, the secretary will usually do his or her best to accommodate you. Sometimes it is easier and quicker to see one of the other chiropractors in the clinic instead. At the time of making the initial appointment you will probably be asked at least for your full name and address and telephone number.

Will your family doctor refer you to a chiropractor?

Whether or not your general practitioner or family doctor refers you to a chiropractor depends almost entirely on the individual doctor, and whether that doctor knows, or is acquainted with the work of, a local chiropractor. In the UK, general practitioners can refer their patients to a chiropractor, or any other therapist, but in doing so they retain the ultimate responsibility for the welfare of the patient while he or she is under that therapist's care. For this reason, it is understandable that the doctor will want to feel confident when referring the patient to another therapist. Very often the doctor may not refer a patient directly to a chiropractor, but may hint that this is what the patient should do.

In the United States, there is still some resistance from family doctors toward chiropractic therapy; many of them are still looking for more research and more proof that chiropractic works. However, there has been a recent softening of attitude and referral is becoming more common – although whether or not a medical practitioner can refer you depends upon the legislation in the state where you live.

If a patient does go to a chiropractor by referral from a doctor, the chiropractor usually keeps the doctor informed about the findings, diagnosis and treatment. If the chiropractor knows that the doctor is open minded towards the treatment, she is usually more than willing to keep the doctor up to date with any progress.

However, if the doctor is vehemently against alternative therapies such as chiropractic – and some still are – then it would be a waste of time and energy to write to him or her. But of course, if the chiropractor diagnoses a condition that cannot be treated by chiropractic therapy, the patient would be referred back to the doctor when necessary, with an accompanying letter, whether or not the doctor appreciates it. It is, after all, the health of the patient that is ultimately of the greatest importance.

What are the likely costs of treatment?

Consultation, treatment and X-ray costs depend to some extent on where the clinic is situated. There are no standard national charges, so a chiropractor's fees tend to vary with the area. In the UK, for example, the charges are usually significantly higher in London than elsewhere. If cost is a problem it may be worth shopping around to find someone.

In the United States, the story is much the same. Costs

depend on local conditions, the number of times you have to attend, competition and so on. There are no fixed rates, but it is usual practice to charge separately for any X-rays that are taken. Medical insurance to cover the costs of chiropractic treatment can be arranged with any of the usual insurers.

Finally, remember that you are making a long-term choice. Ideally, find a practitioner that suits you and stay with her; the more she learns about you, the quirks of your body, the occupational hazards of your job and hobbies, the more helpful she can be, whether it is in an emergency or in a body maintenance programme specific to your needs.

There should be no difficulty in finding a chiropractor to suit you. If you don't find the first practitioner you meet sympathetic, try again.

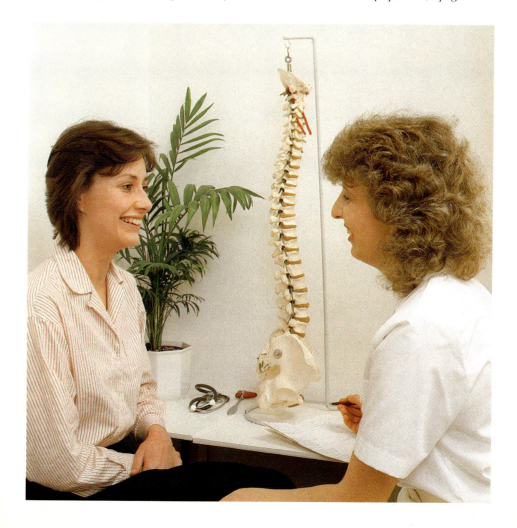

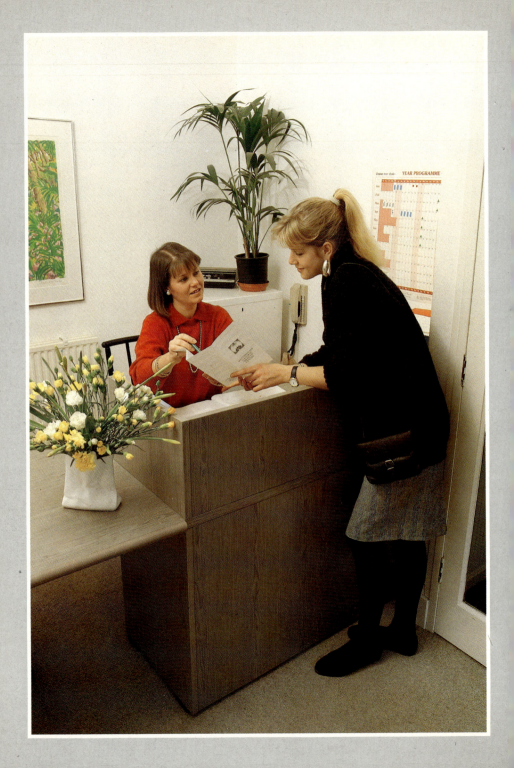

9

USEFUL INFORMATION

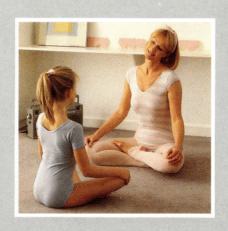

Acute   Used to describe pain or disease that comes on rapidly, usually lasting for a relatively short time.

Adhesion   Membranes sticking together as a result of inflammation, often binding together moving surfaces such as those of JOINTS.

Allergy   An abnormally strong immunity reaction or hypersensitivity, often to everyday substances such as pollen, dust and food.

Aneurysm   A bulge at a weak spot in the wall of an artery.

Angina pectoris   A severe pain in the chest which may radiate down the arms; caused by shortage of oxygen in the heart muscle.

Arthritis   Inflammation of a joint with pain and restriction of movement.
   Osteoarthritis is a degenerative disease of larger JOINTS such as the hip and knee. Rough bone deposits gradually replace CARTILAGE at the joint surfaces.
   Rheumatoid arthritis characterized by chronic painful swelling and distortion of the smaller joints such as the hands.

Asthma   Difficulty in breathing (especially breathing out) due to narrowing of the lung bronchioles (small air passages) and accompanied by wheezing. May be caused by allergy, infection, or emotional disturbances.

Bacterium   A very small living organism (larger than a virus) which can live in animal or vegetable tissue. Bacteria may be benign (such as those that inhabit the human intestines) or harmful.

Biomechanics   The mechanical bases of the biological processes of the body, especially muscular activity; the study of these processes.

Bronchitis   Inflammation of the small air passages in the lungs. It may be ACUTE (brought on by viral or bacterial infection) or chronic – an ongoing inflammation that results in the eventual destruction of lung tissue.

Bursa   A pocket of tissue lined with synovial membrane, as in JOINTS. Bursae reduce friction in areas where tendons or ligaments move over bone.

Bursitis   Inflammation of a bursa, usually by repeated pressure or friction. It often results from repeated actions carried out in particular jobs or hobbies, eg housemaid's knee, tennis elbow.

Cartilage   Gristle; smooth, tough tissue which covers the moving surfaces of JOINTS. When we are born, most of our bones are still cartilage. This allows us to grow, and when we reach full size only a small amount of cartilage remains at the end of each bone. In arthritis, it is this cartilage that becomes rough and eroded rather than smooth.
   The fibrocartilage that sandwiches the vertebrae of the

spine is not the same as joint cartilage, but thick, tough, fibrous tissue.

Chronic   Used to describe pain or disease that affects a person over a long period of time.

Constipation   Failure of waste matter in the large intestine to find its way to the rectum and/or failure of a bowel movement more or less regularly to completely empty the rectum.

Cystitis   Inflammation of the bladder, usually due to bacterial infection. The symptoms are the frequent passing of urine accompanied by a painful burning sensation.

Diathermy   A process used to treat painful, inflamed and stiff joints and muscles. Heat is produced in the tissues by a high frequency electric current.

Diarrhoea   Frequent and often uncontrollable passage of watery bowel motions.

Dysfunction   Failure of an organ or system to function normally.

Dyspepsia   Indigestion.

Flexion   The movement of bending a JOINT (as opposed to extension, or stretching).

Fibrositis   Ill-defined pain in and around muscles, often restricting movement.

Foramen   Hole or passage through a bone or other structure. The spinal nerves leaving the backbone run through the intervertebral foramen.

Fracture   A broken bone. There are several types: a *greenstick fracture* is a partial break in a child's bones; a *simple fracture* is a break with little displacement of the bone and no open wound; in a *compound fracture* the break is exposed through an open skin wound; a *complicated fracture* causes damage to other organs or nerves; in a *comminuted fracture* the bone is splintered.

Frozen shoulder   Stiff and painful shoulder, probably caused by BURSITIS.

Gall bladder   Small 'bag' attached to the underside of the liver, used to store bile.

Groin   Junction of the thigh muscles with those of the belly wall; the groove where each thigh joins the trunk.

Hamstring muscles   The group of muscles at the back of the thigh which flex the knee and help to extend the hip.

Hyperactivity   Overactive behaviour, most commonly applied to children.

Hypermobility   Too much movement (of a JOINT).

Hypomobility   Too little mobility (of a JOINT).

Ilium   The largest part of the hip bone or haunch; part of the PELVIS.

Incontinence   Failure to control the emptying of the bladder or rectum.

Joints   There are two sorts of joints in the human body: mobile or synovial joints and fixed or fibrous joints.
   The body has more synovial joints than fibrous. Where bones meet, the ends of each are enclosed in a thick fibrous capsule which is lined with synovial membrane. This secretes synovial fluid to lubricate the bones as they move against each other.
   Fibrous joints do not allow movement between bones. The bones of the skull are bonded together with fibrous tissue.

Ligament   Fibrous band between two bones at a joint. A ligament is flexible but cannot stretch. Ligaments set the limits beyond which movement is impossible. Any intermediate position of a JOINT is held entirely by muscles. If a joint is forced beyond its normal range, the ligament will tear: this is called a sprain.

Lumbago   Persistent dull pain in the small of the back, often associated with SCIATICA.

Lymph   Colourless fluid which is squeezed out from the body's smallest blood vessels, the capillaries. It washes through the body's tissues, flushing out waste matter, cell debris and bacteria, eventually draining into the LYMPHATIC SYSTEM.

Lymphatic system   A one-way network of drainage channels which receives debris laden LYMPH as it washes through the body tissues. At various points in the system, notably the neck, groin and armpit, there are groups of lymph nodes. These filter off the waste matter and destroy it. They also manufacture some of the antibodies and white blood cells which form the body's defence system. Swollen lymph nodes, visible outside the body and often felt as local discomfort are a sign that your body is dealing with an infection by producing more antibodies.

Mastoiditis   Infection and inflammation of the mastoid bone behind the ear; usually follows from middle ear infection and can lead to deafness.

Meningitis   A dangerous condition where the membranes (*meninges*) covering the brain and spinal cord become inflamed due to viral or bacterial infection.

Migraine   A recurring condition of severe headaches usually with dizziness, nausea and impaired vision.

Multiple sclerosis   A chronic condition of the central nervous system in which small areas of the brain and spinal cord degenerate.

Neuralgia   A pain originating in a nerve (eg SCIATICA).

Neurology   The study of nerves and the nervous system and its disorders. Hence neurological – to do with nerves and the nervous system.

GLOSSARY

Oedema Waterlogging of body tissues, resulting in swelling. Caused by excessive tissue fluid loss from the blood through the walls of the tiniest blood vessels, the capillaries.

Osteoporosis Thinning and weakening of the bones, usually in old age, largely due to calcium loss.

Orthopaedics The whole surgery of bones and joints.

Palpitation Increased awareness of the heartbeat, which may beat more forcibly than usual.

Palpation Method of medical examination by gentle touching.

Patella The kneecap. A thick disc of bone set in the tendon of the quadriceps muscle in front of the knee.

Pelvis The strong girdle of bone which gives stability to the lower part of the body. It consists of the *sacrum* (the five fused lowest vertebrae of the spine) and two hip bones. Each hip bone has three parts: the *ischium* or rump; the *ilium* which supports the sides of the abdomen; and at the front the *pubis*. The pubis of each hip meet at the front of the body, and are bound together by tough fibrous tissue.

Plexus A network of veins and nerves.

Referred pain Pain felt in a different part of the body from the originating site of the infection or injury.

Rheumatism Any painful complaint of muscles or joints not due directly to injury or infection (includes ARTHRITIS, FIBROSITIS, gout).

Sciatica Pain arising anywhere along the path of the sciatic nerve – low back, thigh, calf or foot.

Scoliosis Sideways curvature of the spine.

'Slipped disc' (Prolapsed Intervertebral Disc.) A condition where one of the flexible CARTILAGE pads (the intervertebral discs) between adjacent vertebrae bulges and presses on nearby nerve fibres. Pressure on the spinal nerve causes pain and paralysis in the part it supplies – usually the leg.

Spasm Involuntary contraction of a muscle or LIGAMENT, usually sudden and painful. It can be instant or prolonged.

Spondylitis Inflammation of vertebrae. *Ankylosing spondylitis* ('bamboo spine') is related to rheumatoid ARTHRITIS and causes loss of mobility in the JOINTS between the vertebrae.

Spondylolisthesis A partial dislocation of the spine, usually at the fifth lumbar vertebra of the low back. It is the result of a congenital defect of the vertebra.

Spondylosis The process of wear and tear of the spine, normal with increasing age; can cause aching and stiffness.

Subluxation Displacement of the bones in a joint without complete separation or dislocation.

Symptom A physical or mental change indicating the presence of disorder or disease in the body.

Tendon An extremely tough fibrous cord joining a muscle to a bone. The *achilles tendon* – the large tendon behind the ankle, attached to the heel bone – is particularly subject to great stresses.

Tennis elbow   *see* BURSITIS.

Toxin A toxin produced by the body or by bacteria lodged in food or the body which can cause the symptoms of many diseases.

Traction Continuous pull on a limb during treatment.

Trauma Physical or mental injury. Physical trauma (damaged to tissues) can be caused by blows, burns, wounds etc.

Vascular Of vessels, particularly the blood vessels.

Virus A tiny organism which cannot live independently but thrives in host tissue such as the human body where it causes disease.

USEFUL ADDRESSES

National Associations

British Chiropractic Association
Premier House, 10 Greycoat Place,
London SW1P 1SB

European Chiropractors Union
Tony Metcalfe, DC,
19 Strawberry Hill Road, Twickenham,
Middlesex TW1 4QB

American Chiropractic Association
1916 Wilson Blvd, Arlington, Virginia USA 22201

International Chiropractors Association
1901 L. Street, N.W. Suite 800, Washington, DC,
USA 20036

Australian Chiropractors' Association
1 Martin Place, Linden N.S.W. 2778

Canadian Chiropractic Association
290 Lawrence Avenue West, Toronto,
Ontario M5M 1B3

New Zealand Chiropractors' Association
PO Box 2858, Wellington, New Zealand

Training Colleges
Note: *The courses at all of these colleges is a 4-year, full-time course and entrance requirements would be for 3 science 'A' levels or the individual country's equivalent.*

Great Britain
Anglo-European College of Chiropractic
13-15 Parkwood Road, Boscombe,
Bournemouth BH5 2DF

France
French Institute of Chiropractic
44, rue Duhesme, 75018-Paris, France

Australia
Philip Institute of Technology/School of
Chiropractic
Plenty Road, Bundoora, Victoria 3083

Sydney College of Chiropractic
No. 4 Henson Street, Summer Hill, 2130 Sydney

Canada
Canadian Memorial Chiropractic College
1900 Bayview Avenue, Toronto, Ontario,
Canada M4G 3E6

USA
Cleveland Chiropractic College
6401 Rockhill Road, Kansas City, Missouri 64131

Cleveland Chiropractic College LA
590 North Vermont Avenue, Los Angeles,
California 90004

Life Chiropractic College
1269 Barclay Circle, Marietta, Georgia 30060

Logan College of Chiropractic
1851 Schoettler Road, Box 100
Chesterfield, Missouri 63017

Los Angeles College of Chiropractic
16200 E. Amber Valley Drive Box 1166, Whittier,
California 90609

National College of Chiropractic
200 East Roosevelt Road, Lombard, Illinois 60148

New York Chiropractic College
Post Office Box 167, Glen Head, New York 11545

Northwestern College of Chiropractic
2501 West 84th Street, Bloomington,
Minnesota 55431

Palmer College of Chiropractic
1000 Brady Street, Davenport, Iowa 52803

Palmer College of Chiropractic-West
1095 Dunford Way, Sunnyvale, California 94087

Texas Chiropractic College
5912 Spencer Highway, Pasadena, Texas 77505

Western States Chiropractic College
2900 N.E. 132 Avenue, Portland, Oregon 97230

FURTHER READING

Chiropractic

Nathanial Altman
The Chiropractic Alternative – a spine owner's Guide
J P Tarcher Inc (USA) 1981

Anthea Courtenay
Chiropractic for Everyone
Penguin 1987

Scott Haldemann, DC, PhD, MD
Modern Developments in the Principles and Practice of Chiropractic
Appleton Century Crofts 1980

Merrijoy Kelner, Oswald Hall, Ian Coulter
Chiropractors – do they help?

Lewis Brooks (UK), 1987/Fitzhenry and Whiteside (Canada) 1980

Lawrence Klein and Sharon Meyer
Chiropractic: an International Bibliography
Iowa 1976

Robert A Leach, AA, DC, FICC
The Chiropractic Theories – A Synopsis of Scientific Research
Williams and Wilkins 1986, Baltimore, Ohio

Susan Moore
Alternative Health: Chiropractic
Optima, London 1988

D D Palmer
The Science, Art and Philosophy of Chiropractic
Portland, Oregon 1910

Arthur G Schofield, DC
Chiropractic
Thorsons 1977

Chiropractic in New Zealand – Report of the Commission of Enquiry 1979
Wellington (NZ) 1979

General

Boston Women's Health Collective (Angela Phillips and Jill Rakusen eds)
Our Bodies, Our Selves
Penguin/Boston Women's Collective 1978

Fritjof Capra
The Turning Point
Fontana, London 1983

Dr S J Fulder
A Handbook of Complementary Medicine
Coronet Books, London 1984

Ivan Illich
Limits to Medicine: Medical Nemesis
Calder & Boyars
London 1976; Penguin 1977

Brian Inglis and Ruth West
The Alternative Health Guide
Michael Joseph/Mermaid, London 1983

Leslie K. Kaslof (ed.)
Holistic Dimensions in Healing: A Resource Guide
Doubleday, New York 1978

Gerald Kogan (ed.)
Your Body Works: A Guide to Health, Energy and Balance
Transform, Berkeley, California 1980

E K Ledermann
Good Health through Natural Therapy
Kogan Page, London 1976

Patrick C Pietroni
Holistic Medicine: Old Map, New Territory
British Journal of Holistic Medicine, vol 1, London 1984

Richard Totman
Social Causes of Illness
Souvenir Press, London 1979

Michael van Straten
The Natural Health Consultant
Ebury Press, London 1987

INDEX

INDEX

INDEX

ACKNOWLEDGMENTS

The publishers would like to thank the following organizations and
individuals for their kind permission to reproduce the
illustrations in this book:

Mary Evans Picture Library: 126, 127, 130, 139 **Susan Griggs
Agency/Sandra Lousada**: 24 below **Octopus Publishing Group/Picture
Library**: Chris Harvey/82, 114 left, 114 right, 115 left, 115 right, 118, 119;
Sandra Lousada/33, 111 **Popperfoto**: 47 **Ann Ronan Picture Library**: 137
Science Photo Library: 42 below, 66, 122 right, 123, 125 **Tony Stone
Associates**: 34, 67 **Thorsons Publishing Group Ltd**: 7, 46 **Transworld
Features**: 117 **John Watney**: 94 **Wellcome Institute Library, London**: 134,
135 **Zefa**: 26, 31, 32, 36, 70 left, 70 right, 81, 105, 106, 109, 110

The following photographs were specially taken by Peter Chadwick: 2,
6, 10, 11, 19 below, 23 above, 29 above, 29 below, 35 left, 35 right, 38, 39, 44,
45, 48, 52, 54, 55, 56, 57, 60, 61, 63 top left, 63 top right, 63 bottom, 73, 74, 75,
77, 78, 84, 85, 89, 90, 91 above, 92, 93, 97, 98, 99, 100, 102, 116, 143, 144, 145,
149, 150

Our thanks to the **Westminster Natural Health Centre, London**
for their help with these photographs.

Illustrations by Elaine Anderson

Editor Viv Croot   **Art Editor** Alyson Kyles
Coordinating Editor Camilla Simmons   **Designer** Malcolm Smythe
Production Alyssum Ross   **Picture research** Angie Grant